"Janet Thompson has provided a much needed resource for those ... creating our families. Now the mom of two after seven pregnanc... would have comforted me and perhaps helped me discover what... blessing to read and a comfort."

—**MARDIE CALDWELL** COAP, founder of Lifetime Adoption Center and Adoptive Mom
www.LifetimeAdoptionFoundation.org

"Each well thought out chapter of Janet's book captures the journey of infertility through the real life experiences of her two daughters and other real life couples. Janet's book is well written and easy to follow."

—**VALERIE GELB**, LMFT, www.valeriegelb.com

"Janet, her own miracle daughter Kim, and co-endometriosis sufferer and step-daughter Shannon, offer a unique combination of personal journal letters to God along with Janet's words of mentorship."

—**JENNIFER SAAKE**, author of *Seeking God's Heart in the Midst of Infertility, Miscarriage & Adoption Loss*

"Swimming through all the unknowns of infertility, this book provides you with a tangible reminder that you are not alone. When you are striving to conceive, infertility often brings unrest, frustration, and disappointment. The reminder of God's promises will bring peace to your unrest. The journaling and insights will combat your frustration with a fresh outlook. The encouragement of others' stories comfort your disappointment. No matter where you end up, one of the best gifts you can give yourself along your journey with infertility is peace in your heart."

—**MEGAN FABIAN**, Snowflakes Program Manager, Nightlight Christian Adoptions, www.nightlight.org

"Janet Thompson's *Dear God, Why Can't I Have a Baby?* is a companion to guide and comfort you wherever you are in your infertility or faith journey. Insights from couples who have experienced infertility, pertinent Scriptures, and meaningful prayers encourage you as you seek and find God's purpose in your journey toward parenthood. A practical resource for couples who are trying to have a baby and for family and friends who want to encourage couples dealing with infertility."

—**DEBBIE TAYLOR WILLIAMS**, Christian speaker, author of *The Plan A Woman in a Plan B World: What to Do When Life Doesn't Go According to Plan.*

"As someone who is currently dealing with infertility, *Dear God, Why Can't I have a Baby?* addresses it all. It tenderly guides you through emotional and spiritual questions, grieving, physical alternatives, and adoption to help you and your husband create a family plan together. You'll be encouraged as Janet ...ompson, her daughters, and others vulnerably share their intimate insights and struggles trying to ...t pregnant and the different paths they chose toward parenthood. Personalized love notes from God ...d heartfelt prayers will lift your heart and remind you that you aren't alone in your journey. Janet also ...vides places for you to journal your personal story toward parenthood by writing love letters back to ...d. I highly recommend this book for all want to be parents!"

—**LEANN WEISS-RUPARD**, best-selling author of *Hugs*, founder of Encouragement Company

A Companion Guide
for Couples on the
Infertility Journey

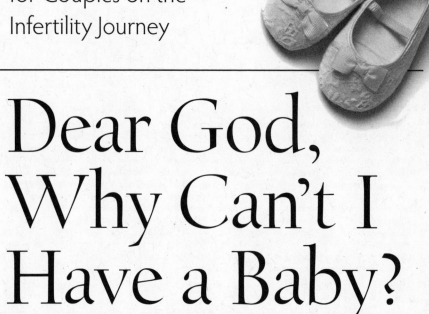

Dear God,
Why Can't I
Have a Baby?

JANET THOMPSON

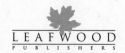

LEAFWOOD
PUBLISHERS

DEAR GOD, WHY CAN'T I HAVE A BABY?

A Companion Guide for Couples on the Infertility Journey

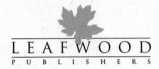

LEAFWOOD
P U B L I S H E R S

First edition

ISBN 978-0-89112-274-6
LCCN 2011000334

Printed in the United States of America

LIBRARY OF CONGRESS CATALOGING-IN-PUBLICATION DATA
Thompson, Janet, 1947-
 Dear god, why can't I have a baby? : a companion guide for couples on the infertility journey / Janet Thompson. -- 1st ed.
    p. cm.
Includes bibliographical references and index.
ISBN 978-0-89112-274-6 (alk. paper)
1. Infertility--Religious aspects--Christianity. I. Title.
RC889.T53 2011
616.6'92--dc22

                                                      2011000334

Cover design by Thinkpen Design, Inc.
Interior text design by Sandy Armstrong

Leafwood is an imprint of
Abilene Christian University Press
1626 Campus Court
Abilene, Texas 79601

1-877-816-4455
www.leafwoodpublishers.com

11 12 13 14 15 16 / 7 6 5 4 3 2 1

DEDICATION

*To my daughters, Kimberly and Shannon, for allowing
God to use your pain and blessings to his glory.
You are beautiful, godly women, and I love you dearly.*

Contents

Acknowledgements

At some time in life, everyone cries out to God, "Why?" The brave men and women sharing their stories in this book all asked, "Dear God, Why Can't I Have a Baby?" If you picked up this book, you or a loved one are asking the same question. To help provide answers of encouragement and hope, Mommies- and Daddies-in-Waiting share their heartache openly and vulnerably.

Kimberly and Toby, you continue to graciously allow me to share God at work in your life and family. You've seen the hand of God perform miracles. Never stop telling your story.

Shannon and Dan, the journey has been long and laced with pain and joy, but you kept the faith and God was gracious. Thank you for reliving those dark times to shed light on God's glorious plans.

Every couple who bravely and boldly shared your story to enlighten and assure other couples that God is good and his love endures forever. Bless your family and your message.

My husband, Dave, helpmate, proofreader, office manager, dishwasher, and all the many hats you wear when I'm entrenched in a deadline. Your support and love help me answer the "Whys" in our life. You always remind me to trust God.

My dear friend and walking buddy, Sharron Pankhurst, who prays for me as I angst about my writing projects in our early morning walks, and freely offers her editing gift as a labor of love to my projects. I thank God for you and our friendship.

Steve Laube, my agent who never gave up on this project. We did it. Thank you for keeping the faith in me and the message of this book.

Leafwood Publishers for appreciating the need for a book that speaks to the millions of couples who ask God for a baby. Thank you for your support and vision for how God will use *Dear God, Why Can't I Have a Baby?*.

Foreword

An Infertility Testimony of Hope

By Drew Cline, Christian recording artist

I've always loved children. Being the youngest of four in my family, I never had the experience of a baby sister or brother to play with or torment. Since I'm a nurturer, I loved holding and playing with babies anytime I could be around them. I couldn't wait to be a father. I'm a very relational person, and my greatest dream in life was to have a family of my own.

When my wife Lori and I married in 1994, like most young couples, we thought we would take a couple of years of wedded bliss and then start the process of having babies and our family. I remember us making plans for a boy or girl—choosing cute names, and creating perfect images of nurseries and strollers and all things children—as if we had some control over those things.

Having a family wasn't my only dream. I also dreamed of being a contemporary Christian music artist. Like most kids, I dreamed of huge crowds, loud music, and making records. I worked with passion to become that artist and to follow my dream, and in many ways I saw it come true. I traveled on the road full-time shortly after getting married, performing nearly a thousand concerts in three years, and Lori followed her own dream of being a radio DJ and working with artists. Before we knew it, we had been married over eight years and still had no children. Our busy schedules and career-chasing kept us from worrying too much about it, and we were young. We thought we would have plenty of time.

As time rolled on, we knew there was a problem and went to a few specialists. Lori had a surgical procedure to help with her endometriosis, and I remember the doctor saying, "You'll be fertile Myrtle now!" A few years later, we still had not conceived, and we hadn't moved any further toward finding out the source of the problem. Lori was given a clean bill of health and so was I—still no children. We continued to follow our careers and dreams, but we found that we were becoming bitter and unbelievably sensitive about children. Most of our friends already had one or two and made comments about how they couldn't even sit too close to each other without getting pregnant. Those kinds of comments, and even story-lines in movies or TV shows that dealt with abortion or babies, were unbelievably difficult for us.

We began to notice our dreams and careers felt shallow. We so deeply longed for children. As we wrestled with what steps to take in fertility, we realized that Lori was struggling with even the idea of being a mommy. Her parents had divorced after seventeen years of marriage, and for some reason, Lori felt children had something to do with that. We had a pretty big argument about where we were, how old we were getting, and whether or not we were going to try anymore. Lori had begun to worry about what kind of mom she would be and whether having children would affect our marriage negatively. After all, she hadn't seen it work well. We were stuck. I wanted to move on toward discovering what was keeping us from getting pregnant, and she was paralyzed with fear of what might happen if we did.

We went to see a dear friend and Christian counselor who helped us and encouraged Lori. After a few sessions, we were seeing truth and growing hope-ful of what having a baby would be like. We made an appointment with a fertility clinic and began the very difficult process of assisted fertility. I'll never forget the time in the middle of that process—after we had had two failed attempts at artifi-cial insemination, feeling embarrassed as if we were lab rats—I said to Lori, "This should be done at home where we can love on each other in the privacy of our own home and marriage, not in some cold clinical test tube. Does God not think we'll make good parents?" To which my precious wife responded, "It takes more love to walk through this process, more sacrifice, more commitment." I began to cry and remember why we were walking this road.

We finally moved forward with in vitro fertilization (IVF), and though Lori is deathly afraid of needles, we made it through. We conceived! On January 25, 2007, we gave birth to our beautiful little girl, Daisy Joy. Daisy has been such an incredible gift from the Lord, and there's not a day that goes by that we don't thank him for her.

During the IVF process, we had three embryos that continued to grow and be viable for implant. Two were implanted when we conceived with Daisy, one was lost, and one was frozen. About a year ago, we decided to go and get our little "snowflake" and start the process of praying and talking with the fertility clinic about what steps should be taken. We had a busy summer in 2009, and though we had hoped to try the implant in June, we didn't actually make time in our schedule until September. We found ourselves waiting for Lori's cycle to begin so we could communicate with the clinic and start the process. We realized that she was nine days late, and Lori mentioned to me that she was a little confused as to why. We had a test that night, and the next day discovered we were pregnant on our own. I was convinced this was a nearly immaculate conception . . . God was involved, no doubt!

On May 25, 2010, we gave birth to our second little girl, Jovie May! We will try to retrieve our little "snowflake" next year sometime. God is so good and has been present with us through it all. There were so many times that it felt like we were in a desert, and surely he wasn't listening, but "he's never left us or forsaken us." His timing is perfect and he is always good. He allows us to walk through some diffi-cult seasons in life, but we are never alone. The question is: Do we trust him? This is his story he's writing, not ours.

It's been such a blessing to write our story for you and remember God's faith-fulness. I'm in tears this morning, so blessed to be a father and a husband.

Blessings on your efforts to care for those wounded and lost in this dark place of infertility.

—*Drew Cline*

Drew has served the church for twenty years on staff or as a guest musical artist. He was the lead singer for NewSong in 2006–2007, recording their Dove Award-nominated "The Christmas Hope" project and has released four of his own solo projects. "Way of Life" was released in 2007, and he is currently working on his fifth project, which he hopes to give away for different partner charities at his website. Drew has been married over sixteen years to his beautiful wife Lori and has two precious girls, Daisy Joy and Jovie May. They live in Franklin, TN. For more information, please go to www.drewcline.com.

Preface

Our Family's Infertility Story

"Janet, you'll never have a baby. Your ovaries look like those of a ninety-year-old woman."

I was sitting on the doctor's exam table, extending my left hand to show him my new engagement ring. I protested in shock, "But I'm engaged!"

"You'll have to tell your fiancé you probably will never have children. If he *really* loves you, he'll understand and still want to marry you," the doctor replied.

This dismal prognosis occurred at my post-op visit following an emergency operation for suspected appendicitis, which turned out to be a ruptured ovarian cyst. The surgeon on call the night of my surgery, who happened to be an OB-GYN, was now pronouncing pregnancy a virtual impossibility after seeing my "shriveled up and cyst-covered" ovaries. I was twenty-one, a college senior, and newly engaged—and my world was over. I couldn't have children—the dream of every little girl who ever played house.

Even as a teenager, my happily-ever-after vision had seemed tenuous as my friends started menstruation and I anxiously awaited my turn. I waited and waited. Finally, in my junior year of high school, an endocrinologist determined that my internal female organs weren't properly developed. He prescribed a regimen of pills and shots, to which I faithfully adhered until, at eighteen, it was time to leave for college.

Several months after starting college, my long-awaited passage into womanhood arrived. What a pleasant surprise and relief! That was until monthly cramps had me doubling over and bedridden with unbelievable pain. I didn't relish this phase of being a woman, but I knew it was essential for having a baby, someday.

Now this doctor was telling me that in five years I had gone from having underdeveloped female organs to ones resembling those of a ninety-year-old woman. Doctors were supposed to fix things. Had something gone wrong with the endocrinologist's treatment? I was stunned. Numb. How would I tell my fiancé that he might want to reconsider his marriage proposal?

In announcing my sorry plight, the doctor didn't use the word *infertility*, and I'm not sure I would have understood the term if he had. But he did use words I clearly understood—even though I didn't want to—I wasn't *ever* going to have a baby!

In those days, the more frequent terms for infertility were *barren*, *not able to have children*, or *childless*. Seldom were these "conditions" mentioned in public. If a couple was childless, they must not want children. People didn't openly discuss such private issues.

My mother gave birth to me six days before her first wedding anniversary, but having a second baby wasn't as easy for my parents. I was an "only child" for six years before they finally had my sister. Today, we call that condition *secondary infertility*.

When I told my fiancé the doctor's prognosis, he said his mother was adopted and that adoption was a fine solution. I was grateful for his reaction, but I secretly held on to the notion that we would have a baby. While I understood the doctor's words—that I would be one of "those unfortunate childless women"—I didn't accept his proclamation. I decided this wouldn't happen to me: I *was* going to have a baby. I'm not sure if my youthful optimism evolved from naïveté, ignorance, arrogance, denial, or refusal to accept one doctor's opinion (albeit a doctor who had examined my deteriorating ovaries). Still, I held on to the dream of having a baby.

My fiancé and I did marry the day after we graduated from college. In the early years of marriage, it was a relief not to worry about getting pregnant because we were both starting new careers. But I gazed longingly at the couple next door who were expecting their first baby. I wondered if *my* tummy would ever bulge with a new life.

Three years into marriage, the unexplainable happened. Like Sarah in the Bible, who laughed at the thought of getting pregnant at age ninety, I was laughing at the doctor who said my "ninety year old" ovaries would never produce a child. I was pregnant! The Lord's words to Sarah's husband, Abraham, echoed in my mind. "Is anything too hard for the LORD?" (Gen. 18:14). When I gave birth to my daughter, Kimberly, my mother called her a "little miracle." At the time, I resented her making such a big deal about my *unusual* pregnancy—I longed to be "normal." As I grew in my faith, I was able to appreciate God's mercy and grace, which blessed me with the miracle of Kim's life.

Normal was short-lived. When Kim was six months old, I had a pulmonary embolism, and doctors warned me not to get pregnant for eighteen months. Unfortunately, when Kim was two, her father and I separated and later divorced. I didn't remarry until I was forty-five, and my husband Dave had three children from a previous marriage, so we had a full house. I never had the opportunity to find out whether I was capable of having more children.

As my "miracle baby" Kim was growing up, she would often pat her tummy and announce, "Someday there's going to be a baby in there." I'd smile and nod my head in agreement, while my heart was pleading, *Oh Lord, please let it be so. My mom and I may have passed down something genetically to Kim. Please let my baby have a baby.*

Then the fear lurking at the fringes of my mind and heart was justified when Kim married Toby, and they began trying to have a baby. They had waited three years, thinking Kim would go off birth control pills and quickly get pregnant—right on schedule. But as the months turned into years, and she didn't ovulate or have a period, the concern mounted. So began their infertility journey.

When my husband Dave and I married, two of his children, Shannon and Sean, came to live with us. Shannon and I endured the same monthly pain caused by endometriosis. We shared pain pills and the heating pad and understood each other's "time of the month." We both had laparoscopies to surgically remove endometrial scar tissue to help ease the pain, and in Shannon's case, reduce her risk of infertility. Unfortunately, infertility later became a reality for her.

In *Dear God, Why Can't I Have a Baby?* Kim and Shannon invite you along on their journeys with infertility and God. Their medical issues and resolutions may differ from yours, but you'll resonate with their hearts.

Kim's husband, Toby, and Shannon's husband, Dan, graciously support their wives in sharing our family's story of hurt, pain, sadness, and gladness. Infertility affects the entire family. When Dave and I married, we quickly accepted each other's children into our home and hearts, so I refer to my three stepchildren as "my" children, and Dave does the same with Kim. For clarity, Kim is my birth daughter, and Shannon is my gift daughter by marriage.

Kim, Shannon, and I hope and pray that *Dear God, Why Can't I Have a Baby?* provides a source of hope and encouragement as the three of us walk beside you on your infertility journey. Difficult life journeys seem less scary and forbidding with a friend next to you. Ecclesiastes 4:9 and 12 confirm, "Two are better than one," and, "A cord of three strands is not quickly broken"—the Lord, you, and us.

On the journey with you,
Janet, Kim, and Shannon

Introduction

MY PURPOSE IN WRITING IS SIMPLY THIS: THAT YOU WHO BELIEVE IN
GOD'S SON WILL KNOW BEYOND THE SHADOW OF A DOUBT THAT YOU
HAVE ETERNAL LIFE, THE REALITY AND NOT THE ILLUSION.
—1 John 5:13 *The Message*

My daughters, Kim and Shannon, and I have a window into your feelings and pain.
We want to walk beside you as only friends who have been in your shoes can. Our
desire is to mentor and encourage you from our experiences and to wrap you in God's
goodness, peace, and love. While we may not know your name, we know your heart.

Dear God, Why Can't I Have a Baby? is a companion to guide and comfort you
wherever you are in your infertility or faith journey. We trust this book will also be
an oasis of solace and comfort from God's Word as you seek and find God's purpose
in your journey toward parenthood. For each of you, God's plan and purpose will
be different and unique, but rest assured, he does have a plan. Nothing happens by
accident in a believer's life. If we know God's son Jesus as our personal Savior, we
know that God "causes all things to work together for good to those who love God,
to those who are called according to His purpose" (Rom. 8:28 NASB).

Where to Begin?

This is your book to use in ways that serve you best. The chapters start at the beginning of the infertility journey and progress through decisions, treatments, emotions,
things to remember, things to forget, and tools to help you maintain your sanity.

Kim's and Shannon's stories start in Chapter One and progress through
the book in Dear God journal entries. Stories from contributing Mommies- and
Daddies-in-Waiting, and other quoted resources, compliment the girls' entries. If
you're just beginning to sense infertility issues or have been recently diagnosed,
start at the beginning of the book or turn to the topic touching your life today.

For those of you entrenched in the infertility battle or who may have struggled
with it many years ago, let this book help you work through feelings of grief, sorrow,
hurt, anger, emptiness, and brokenness and also help you remember the joys and
blessings. Each chapter is divided into several topics with the following subsections:

The Topic Title—Followed by a quote and a Scripture

Dear God Journal from Kim or Shannon—Janet's daughters share their infertility journeys.

A Mommy- or Daddy-in-Waiting Shares—Contributing couples share their infertility journeys. All stories are true and shared with permission, but some names have been changed.

Janet's Mentoring Moment—Helpful tips and encouragement from the author.

God's Love Letter to You—Personalized, paraphrased Scripture.

Couple's Prayer—A prayer for husband and wife to pray together.

Your Letter to God—Encouraging prompts and a place to journal your story.

Take this book with you to doctors' appointments, tests, procedures, ultrasounds, the hospital, adoption agencies, the adoption lawyer's offices, and wherever the twists and turns of your infertility journey take you. With your book in hand:

- Read. Take notes. Journal.
- Write questions to ask and then record the answers.
- Read an encouraging story from another couple dealing with infertility.
- Note something to remember about a fellow infertility sojourner you meet along the way.
- Receive God's comfort from his Love Letter to You.

Journaling

My vision for *Dear God, Why Can't I Have a Baby?* is for the book to be a safe place to document an epic time in your life. Whether you've journaled regularly for years or this is your first time, there is freedom and healing in expressing your thoughts and feelings in writing.

Shannon commented that journaling and writing her Dear God entries for this book was cathartic. I found the same thing to be true when I wrote about my breast cancer experience in *Dear God, They Say It's Cancer*. At the end of each chapter, there's space for journaling your own Dear God entries, and you may want to write more in a separate journal.

Healing often happens when we talk about what's bothering us—or write about it. Think of journaling as writing a letter to God. Not everyone understands, but God always understands, and he is eager to hear from you. Regardless of your faith, you matter to God. God will fill the pages by nudging you toward helpful things to write. Maybe he will help you remember a good time or a different way of looking at a person who unintentionally said something hurtful. Some days you'll write pages; other days you won't feel like writing more than a sentence.

Your journaling is personal. Don't feel you have to share it with anyone. However, as God did with Kim, Shannon, and the couples who share their stories in this book, God might provide opportunities for you to mentor others with the wisdom and encouragement you've learned along the journey.

Kim's and Shannon's Dear God journal entries are a compilation of reflections back to their early days of infertility as well as discussions of current feelings about this struggle. You may want to follow their format and combine looking back at past experiences with descriptions of what you're currently encountering. During the heat of the battle, when you're fighting the daily barrage of decisions or assaults to your body, you often don't feel like doing or thinking anything. However, when the crisis subsides, you'll wish you had written things down.

The best part about journaling is that God is ready to receive your words with a faithful, listening ear. He can take it all: the good, the bad, and the ugly. He beckons, "Come to me, all you who are weary and burdened, and I will give you rest. Take my yoke upon you and learn from me, for I am gentle and humble in heart, and you will find rest for your souls. For my yoke is easy and my burden is light" (Matt. 11:28–30).

Journaling Tips

If you need some guidance to get started writing your thoughts, try the following ideas:

- Pray before you start.
- Write your heart. Let your pen flow with thoughts and feelings.
- Don't worry about grammar, spelling, or sounding articulate or spiritual.
- Think of journaling as writing a letter to God or as a written conversation with God.
- Date your entries.
- Reflect on Kim's or Shannon's Dear God journal entries or comment on one of the Mommy- or Daddy-in-Waiting stories or Janet's Mentoring Moments. Consider how it applies to you.

- Don't feel confined to answering the thought-provoking questions at the end of each chapter under Your Letter to God.
- Develop abbreviations and symbols that only you understand.
- When it hurts, talk about it. When you're mad, cry out—God can take it.
- Express good things, too, and make sure to write on the days where everything does seem better.
- Journal while waiting in examination or treatment rooms, when you can't sleep, during bed rest or hospitalizations, or during quiet times with God.
- Let this book be your constant companion.
- Don't worry if the pen seems too heavy—journaling shouldn't make you feel guilty. Reading God's Love Letter to You might provide more comfort at the moment.
- Record prayer requests and God's answers in the Prayer & Praise Journal, page 272.

Personalizing and Praying Scripture

Dear God, Why Can't I Have a Baby? can be read as a devotional—a study of how God's Word, the Bible, applies to your life—specific to your infertility issues. The Bible provides the guidance, direction, peace, and answers you seek. It's "A manual for living, for learning what's right and just and fair; To teach the inexperienced the ropes and give our young people a grasp on reality. There's something here also for seasoned men and women, still a thing or two for the experienced to learn—Fresh wisdom to probe and penetrate, the rhymes and reasons of wise men and women. Start with GOD" (Prov. 1:3–7 *The Message*).

The Bible is your personal guide for life. *Nothing else* will fill the deep need and hole in your heart except God and his Word. Often in the Couple's Prayer section, you'll pray personalized, paraphrased Scriptures. *The Message* adapts well to praying because it's a paraphrase of the Bible in modern-day language rather than a literal translation. Try praying the following personalized Scripture (Ps. 86:11–12 NLT paraphrased): Lord, teach us your ways, that we may live according to your truth! Grant us purity of heart, so that we may honor you. With all our hearts, we will praise you, O Lord our God. We will give glory to your name forever. Amen.

My prayer for you: May he give you the desire of your heart and make all your plans succeed (Ps. 20:4).

Chapter One

IT'S TIME TO HAVE A BABY

He gives childless couples a family,
gives them joy as the parents of children. Hallelujah!
—Psalm 113:9 *The Message*

We're Ready Now

All my life I looked forward to being a wife and mother. I married at the age of twenty-six, and we tried having a family right away, expecting to get pregnant soon after our wedding. After all, my sister already was pregnant with her third child, and my mother had given birth to six, so I thought getting pregnant would be a snap. I mean, how hard could this be? —Gay Lynne

I'm ready to consummate my marriage.
—Genesis 29:21 *The Message*

Shannon's Journal

Dear God,

God, I've suffered with monthly cramps and ovarian cysts for as long as I can remember. You know I endured two laparoscopy surgeries to remove the endometriosis and went on birth control pills to ease the cyclical pain. Then, at twenty-two and newly engaged to Dan, my doctor recommended having children right away because my "condition" would worsen with time.

But, God, remember the questions I asked you: I still have one more year of college. Shouldn't I wait until after I graduate to get married, like we planned? Should I change my plans? Can I be ready for marriage *and* motherhood?

I'm not sure I stayed still long enough back then to hear your answer. I charged ahead with my own plans. Full of hope, or maybe just wanting to take control, we moved up our wedding date and began trying to get pregnant on our honeymoon. Dan wasn't quite as excited as I was about starting a family so quickly, but he agreed.

Now, as newlyweds, each month that goes by I'm sure I'm pregnant. Each month we're disappointed. I had no idea what a strain the heartache of infertility would be on a new marriage.
Expectantly, Shannon

A Mommy-in-Waiting Shares

It wasn't supposed to be like this. Even when I was a little girl and boys had cooties, I knew that someday I'd grow up, get married, and have children. After all, didn't everyone? As I entered adulthood, everything seemed to be going along fine. I met a wonderful man, got married, and on our honeymoon we had fun discussing what we might name our future children. Later, we bought a house with extra bedrooms for the kids we hoped to have soon. But the years passed, and no children came. No morning sickness, no rounding belly, no baby showers filled with cute little booties and boxes of diapers.[1] —Marlo Schalesky, *Empty Womb, Aching Heart*

Janet's Mentoring Moment

Shannon and Dan explained to my husband Dave and me that, because of Shannon's medical condition, they wanted to move up their wedding date so they could start trying to get pregnant. Pregnancy is a big expectation and undertaking for a new marriage, so we talked about the hard question: What if pregnancy isn't a possibility? Dan and Shannon confirmed their love for each other regardless of what the future held for them concerning children. They were getting married and going for it!

Many couples try to conceive soon after the wedding: *Why wait?* they ask. *Let's start filling the bedrooms in our house as soon as possible.* When "soon" isn't possible, their panicked cry is: *Dear God, why can't I have a baby?*

Maybe you're one of these couples consumed with the desire for a child. Your wedding day is a faint memory in your quest to conceive. You might find it helpful and refreshing to take a breather from trying to get pregnant and enjoy being newlyweds. You're not giving up—you're just taking a break.

God's Love Letter to You

Dear_____ and _____,

I, God, made you male and female to be together. Because of this, a man leaves his father and mother, and in marriage he becomes one flesh with a woman—no longer two individuals, but forming a new unity (Mark 10:6-8 *The Message*, paraphrased).
Creator of marriage, God

Couple's Prayer

Lord, We thank you for creating marriage and for bringing us together as husband and wife. We want to become parents, and the desire of our hearts is to have children. We're trying, but it isn't happening. Please help us understand your plan and timing for our marriage. Show us how to cope with the disappointment of our unfulfilled dream of immediate parenthood. Remind us to enjoy being married. Amen.

OUR MASTER PLAN

From the time I was a young girl, I had a "Master Plan." I assumed some-
day I'd find Mr. Right, marry him, and have his babies.[2]
—Laura Christianson, *The Adoption Decision*

WE HUMANS KEEP BRAINSTORMING OPTIONS AND PLANS,
BUT GOD'S PURPOSE PREVAILS.
—PROVERBS 19:21 *The Message*

Kim's Journal

Dear God,
Most young women think you made us to be mothers—it's a natural part of life. We grow up, graduate, get married, and start a family. My life seemed right on track with that plan. I graduated from college, started a great career, and met the love of my life, Toby. You know, God, that Toby and I both gave our hearts to your Son, Jesus, just a few weeks before we were married, so it seemed life couldn't get any sweeter.

Toby and I decided that before settling down to start a family, we would: buy a house, pay off debts, and travel, and Toby would finish college. Over a three-year period, we checked off everything on our list, culminating with a fabulous trip to Italy.

From the beginning of our relationship, we had talked about having children, but as we completed our "checklist," Toby seemed nervous. He suggested taking a child development class. I reassured him that most people don't know what they're getting into, and there'd never be the "right time." Children are your creation, God. You'd help us face any parenthood challenges. Finally, I convinced Toby we were ready, and he agreed. So when we returned home from Italy, I stopped taking birth control pills. It was time to start a family. "Our plan" was in place.
Planning, Kim

Two Mommies-in-Waiting Share

Our newlywed "Master Plan" included establishing careers as high school teachers, attending graduate school, seeing as much of the world as possible, and purchasing a home. Robert, a math teacher who creates convoluted budgets "just for fun," estimated we would be financially ready to have children after five years of marriage. So, after five years of wedded bliss, we got to work on Project: Baby.[3]
—Laura Christianson

We're control freaks and when we married, we said we would wait five years to have children. So right on plan, we started trying to have a baby at four years and three months. I was so regular, we were sure we would get pregnant right away because that was the plan, right? We had completed college, secured great jobs in the military, traveled, and I had finished active duty and was working as a CPA. Financially stable, we felt we had done everything right. We were on track and moving to the next step—starting our family. Isn't it funny how we almost feel entitled to these things? —Karen

Janet's Mentoring Moment

One Christmas, Dave and I gave our granddaughter, Arianna, a dollhouse that came with a mommy, daddy, baby, and dog. From childhood, most girls fantasize about having a family and being a mother, while boys expect to provide for a family and become a father. Nesting and procreating are nearly universal human drives perceived as God-given rights.

Roles take shape during puberty for making this dream a reality: girls start menstruation, and boys grow hair on their faces. We learn about sex, conception, and reproduction, and that's what we plan to do someday—reproduce. With the advent of birth control, there's a sense of being in charge of our destiny: planned parenthood.

Then when we're ready but our bodies aren't, we start asking God what went wrong. We plead with him to bless our timetable, but God might be saying, "You didn't include me in these plans." Even if you did include God, often the Master's plan differs from our master plan. To revise or create a new plan, go to Making Decisions and Developing a Family Plan, page 255.

God's Love Letter to You

Dear _____ and _____ ,

I know what I'm doing. I have it all planned out—plans to take care of you, not abandon you, plans to give you the future you hope for (Jer. 29:11 *The Message*).

The Master, God

Couple's Prayer

Lord, We're so confused. We feel like we've done everything right, yet still you haven't blessed us with a child. It doesn't seem fair and our hearts are breaking. Help us surrender our will to your will, our plan to your plans for our future. We believe in you, Lord, as we know you believe in us. Our hope is in you. Amen.

ARE WE DOING SOMETHING WRONG?

Robert's brother informed us that all he had to do was look at his wife and she got pregnant. Maybe that was the problem. We just weren't doing it right.[4] —Laura Christianson

When we decided to adopt a baby before having one of our own, my concerned dad asked if we knew how to make a baby! —Lynne

IS NOT MY HOUSE RIGHT WITH GOD? HAS HE NOT MADE WITH ME AN EVER-LASTING COVENANT, ARRANGED AND SECURED IN EVERY PART? WILL HE NOT BRING TO FRUITION MY SALVATION AND GRANT ME MY EVERY DESIRE?
—2 Samuel 23:5

Shannon's Journal

Dear God,

Every month I suspect I might be pregnant, and then it comes—my period. I worry about when to have sex, how often, and whether I'm taking my temperature right. Now I'm starting to wonder, God . . . why aren't I getting pregnant?

I thought it would be OK to jump right into motherhood. After all, my sister-in-law Janel is pregnant, and they just got married! She gets to be a mom—why don't I? I had visions of being new moms and raising our kids together. What happened? I keep thinking my turn is right around the corner. Now a year has passed and, frankly, I'm tired. Tired of trying, tired of timing sex, tired of taking temperatures . . . just tired of it all!

Wearily, Shannon

A Mommy-in-Waiting Shares

With our graduate studies complete, Robert and I had our summers off to travel and relax (I'd heard that relaxing helps you get pregnant). We traveled to Great Britain. No baby. We traveled to Australia. No baby. We traveled to France. No baby. We traveled to Scandinavia. Still no baby. My sisters-in-law, who never traveled, were breeding babies as quickly as rabbits.

It seemed as if everyone but us was either pregnant or had a baby. It seemed as if our Master Plan—or my ovaries, or Robert's sperm—were malfunctioning. "Why is this happening to us?" we questioned. This kind of stuff wasn't supposed to plague healthy, well-educated, financially secure, church-going married couples who were anxious to become parents.

Robert and I did what any healthy, well-educated, financially secure, church-going couple would do in our position: we cried. We fretted. We begged God for a baby.[5] —Laura Christianson

Janet's Mentoring Moment

You might be thinking you're not doing something right—especially when everyone else seems to have baby making figured out. Anxious and panicked, you may try "quick fix" remedies and become even more frustrated when they don't work. I saw an advertisement for a resort featured as "the place to vacation or weekend for couples trying to get pregnant," as if they had the magic formula and all you had to do was get away to their conceiving paradise.

Few couples prepare for infertility—even with a past injury or problem with reproductive organs. You still feel an innate "right" to have a baby. I know I did. Everyone else is having babies, so you will, too. When you're not "expecting" according to your expected time frame, you can fall into the trap of second-guessing yourself. Or others help out with advice. They say you just need to: relax, take a vacation, adopt a child, eliminate stress, try different positions, stand on your head, stay out of hot tubs, change your diet, have sex every day, don't have sex every day, don't try so hard, try harder—often said with a knowing wink of the eye. The implication is that you're creating your own infertility. How frustrating and ignorant those comments are—so don't listen to them and definitely don't say them to yourself or each other.

Char relates that when she and her husband decided later in life to have a child, "One woman from my Bible study, who had a nursing background, said my husband and I should have intercourse every day on days nine through eighteen of my cycle. My OB-GYN advised that would reduce the sperm count, making us *less likely* to get pregnant. So be careful of well-intended 'folk advice,' even from people with medical backgrounds."

Judith C. Daniluk, PhD, author of *The Infertility Survival Guide*, explains:

> The average chance of conceiving in a month for couples having regular intercourse throughout the menstrual cycle, meaning approximately three times per week, is only about 20 percent per cycle when the woman is less than thirty-five years of age. . . . Beyond thirty-five years, the spontaneous conception rate is estimated to decrease each year. Once a woman is forty years or older, the per cycle rate of conception is only 5 percent. . . . So, whether you're at the beginning of the process of dealing with infertility, or you're currently undergoing a number of medicated or unmedicated intrauterine insemination cycles, try not to panic if you don't become pregnant right away.[6]

Bottom line—enjoy each other. God created marital sex for pleasure. Children are only one of the fruits of that pleasure. God also created intercourse as a means of uniting husband and wife into one body. If you're sharing your bodies with each other, you aren't doing anything wrong.

God's Love Letter to You

Dear_____and_____,

Enjoy the wife you married as a young man! Lovely as an angel, beautiful as a rose—don't ever quit taking delight in her body. Never take her love for granted (Prov. 5:18–19 *The Message*)! *Love always, God*

Couple's Prayer

Lord, We're worried and anxious, and it's difficult enjoying our sexual relations with each other because we wonder if we're doing something wrong. Lord, please remove these anxious thoughts and misgivings. As much as we want to have children, we also want to enjoy each other and our marriage. You are our first love, and our spouse is our second love, and nothing can change that. Amen.

WHY CAN'T I HAVE A BABY?

*Lord, this is so unfair! Bearing children is such a run-of-the-mill female
function. I mean, look at all the thousands of stray kittens and puppies!
So why won't you bless me with children?* —Kelly

IF THE LORD IS WITH US, WHY HAS ALL THIS HAPPENED TO US?
—Judges 6:13

Kim's Journal

Dear God,
I'm starting to worry. I've been off the pill for four months, and I haven't had a period. Many people tell me it could take a few months for a cycle to return to normal, so every month we wait for my period to start. Month after month after month. . . .

When I was a teenager, I heard a statistic that one in six women will struggle with infertility. That really bothered me because I hung out with a group of five girls. Something in the pit of my stomach kept telling me I would be that one in six who wouldn't be able to have children. Shortly after high school, my friends started having babies. Again, that gnawing feeling returned as I wondered if you, God, would ever bless me with children.

It just seems that everyone else is so fertile. That is, everyone except my stepsister Shannon and her husband Dan, who are also struggling with infertility. Why God? Why can't we have our heart's desire? Why can't we have a baby?
Questioningly, Kim

Two Mommies-in-Waiting Share

For someone who grew up constantly playing with dolls and babysitting, becoming a mother should have been an easy and natural course to take after getting married at nineteen. My career plans included being a wife and a mom, period. So when my husband and I had been married a couple of years, we decided it was time to start our family.

I had developed cysts on my ovaries at eighteen, but the doctor said the only difficulty endometriosis might cause in getting pregnant was it might take me a little longer. So, we weren't surprised when a few months went by without becoming pregnant. But after several more went by, we decided to consult a doctor. This began a journey of infertility specialists, tests, surgery, and monthly highs of hopes for pregnancy coupled with lows of finding out it didn't occur again this month.

As I watched many of my friends getting pregnant, sometimes for the second or third time, I became bitter and jealous of my friends and even angry with God. All I'd wanted was to get married and raise children. I'd loved children all my life. Why would He not give us a child?[7] —Chris Adams, "My Struggle with Infertility"

Dear God, why can't I have a baby? You told us to be fruitful and multiply, and yet I can't. Your Word says that children are a blessing from you, a gift. Why don't you want to bless *me*, Lord? Why would you give me this desire and not fulfill it? Am I just being selfish for wanting a baby? If you don't want me to have children, Lord, then please change my heart because from now until the day I die, I'll have this longing, this desire, and it will always be the cry of my heart. —Danette

Janet's Mentoring Moment

You're probably questioning God, too. Why isn't he fulfilling your dream of parenthood? Why does he seem to be silent? It's natural to question and maybe even be angry at God for not quickly "fixing" things—the way you want them fixed. As you write your letter to God at the end of this chapter, talk to him about your pain. God weeps and groans with you. This wasn't how he meant life to be; it wasn't supposed to be this hard. His original plan was for us to live happily and peacefully. But sin entered the world through Adam and Eve, and God's heart has been breaking for his people ever since.

The Bible says that God keeps track of each of your tears: "You've kept track of my every toss and turn through the sleepless nights, each tear entered in your ledger, each ache written in your book" (Ps. 56:8 *The Message*). It might help to set an appointment with a pastor at church or a biblical counselor and ask him or her to pray with you to believe and accept that God is a good God and doesn't want you to suffer.

God's Love Letter to You

Dear _____ and _____,

When you call on me, when you come and pray to me, I'll listen. When you come looking for me, you'll find me. Yes, when you get serious about finding me and want it more than anything else, I'll make sure you won't be disappointed. I'll turn things around for you (Jer. 29:12–14 *The Message*, paraphrased).

I love you, God

Couple's Prayer

Heavenly Father, It's hard not to be mad at you. It seems like with the blink of an eye, you could turn all of this around and help us get pregnant. Why are you holding out? Help us be patient and prayerfully wait on your sovereign plan for our family—the plan that we cannot see right now. Restore our hope and faith. Please turn our questions into answers. We know you might not answer the way we expect. Amen.

HOW LONG SHOULD WE TRY BEFORE SEEING A DOCTOR?

Joe and I tried to conceive on our own for four years, then we finally decided to seek medical help. —Jennifer

HOW LONG MUST I WRESTLE WITH MY THOUGHTS AND
EVERY DAY HAVE SORROW IN MY HEART?
—Psalm 13:2

Shannon's Journal

Dear God,

Getting pregnant is harder than I thought, and we're just settling into who takes whose hairbrush and why he hits the snooze button five times before getting up. And more importantly, why doesn't Dan talk to me more or understand me or listen before giving the two-step solution? Who actually lives on a budget? So what if I bounce a few checks? And why is he so obsessed with analyzing our finances with spreadsheets?

God, marriage has been like holding up a mirror and seeing all my faults reflected back daily. I'm just figuring out how to deal with that, and I'm not sure I have it in me to keep on trying to have a baby now. I'm crying from unmet expectations in my marriage, and I'm crying because I can't get pregnant, not even once! This is all too painful. The tests aren't showing anything wrong with my hormones or ovulation.

So what's next? Seeing a specialist? Doing more tests? I'm not ready to go there. I've had enough pain for one year. I can't take any more. I need to heal first. It's time to take a break.

Sadly, Shannon

A Mommy-in-Waiting Shares

We've been trying to get pregnant for three of our six married years. I was diagnosed with polycystic ovary syndrome (PCOS) almost two years ago and went on a few meds to help regulate my blood sugar and endocrine system in hopes that would help conceiving. I haven't tried Clomid or any infertility treatments. At times, the desire to be a mom is overwhelmingly painful! —Heather

Janet's Mentoring Moment

Some couples, like Mandy and her husband, tried to get pregnant for seven years before seeking medical assistance, and another couple waited fourteen years. There's no general "standard" for when to see a doctor except that most doctors won't start checking for infertility until you've been trying without protection for a year or have extenuating medical issues or a history of fertility problems in either of your families.

You may feel at a crossroads, wondering if you should continue trying to get pregnant on your own, talk with a doctor, or focus on your marriage before adding children. The decision as to when to see a doctor includes more considerations than just the medical ones. Shannon and Dan did take a break and worked on their marriage. Shannon later said about this season of their lives, "God did have plans for us: plans to grow us, change us, and bond us. Those plans just didn't include children for another six years."

God's plan may be for you to build a firm and strong marriage foundation *before* adding children to your family. The two of you *are* a family: children expand your family, and they're a lifetime commitment and responsibility. It's important to confirm and affirm that your commitment to each other is for a lifetime—in sickness and in health, for better or worse, fertile or infertile. A child isn't going to heal or help a strained, unstable marriage. It isn't fair to put that expectation on a baby who comes into the world deserving the best from his or her parents.

God's Love Letter to You

Dear_____ and _____,

If you ask me, I will give you wise minds and spirits attuned to my will, and so you'll acquire a thorough understanding of the ways in which I work. Live well for me, your Master, and make me proud of you as you work hard on your marriage. As you learn more and more how I, God, work, I will give you the strength to stick it out over the long haul—not the grim strength of gritting your teeth but the glory-strength I, God, give. It is strength that endures the unendurable and spills over into joy, thanking me, the Father, who makes you strong enough to take part in everything bright and beautiful that I have for you. (Col. 1:9–12 *The Message,* paraphrased)

Praying for you, God

Couple's Prayer

Lord, It's hard to know what to do next. We want to be wise and listen for your guidance. Please give us those times of quiet and unity when we come together in prayer and seek your will and way. Help us know the next step to take, and let us be in agreement about when we should move forward in a different direction. Help our marriage withstand the stress and strain of infertility. Let our love so shine before others that they see your light shining in the midst of our darkness. Amen.

Your Letter to God

Even saying the word "infertility" probably brings you to tears, not to mention thinking of it applying to you. As you consider where to go from here, pour out your pain, confusion, disappointment, discouragement, fears, and frustrations, but don't forget those bright moments, too. Let God know how you're feeling. He's waiting with a listening, compassionate ear.

Dear God,   *Date:*

_____

_____

_____

_____

_____

_____

_____

_____

_____

_____

_____

_____

_____

_____

Chapter Two

MAKING THE DOCTOR'S APPOINTMENT

I HAVE HEARD ALL ABOUT YOU, LORD,
AND I AM FILLED WITH AWE BY THE AMAZING THINGS YOU HAVE DONE.
IN THIS TIME OF OUR DEEP NEED, BEGIN AGAIN TO HELP US,
AS YOU DID IN YEARS GONE BY.
SHOW US YOUR POWER TO SAVE US.
—Habakkuk 3:2 NLT

Where Do We Start?

All my tests are finally finished and we've been given the go-ahead to start trying again.
—Laurell

DON'T LOOK TOO CLOSE FOR BLEMISHES, GIVE ME A CLEAN BILL OF HEALTH.
GOD, MAKE A FRESH START IN ME.
—PSALM 51:9–10 *The Message*

Shannon's Journal

Dear God,

Dan keeps asking if I'm ready to try again. I keep saying another year or two. Well, it's been four, and I still don't feel quite ready. My life has been full of so many good things. We've gone to counseling and our marriage is stronger. We got a dog that we love and nurture; he's truly our child and goes everywhere with us. I've found my career teaching special needs children and enjoyed some dance and acting classes. Dan took drum lessons and played in the worship team at church.

There have been so many good, positive things. God, I'm not sure I want to face the disappointment again. I mean, what if there's something really wrong? What if we can't . . . I can't even say it. I don't even want to think it. Though, I do get excited thinking about having a child.

God, be close. Give me your strength as I embark on this journey. Carry me through whatever awaits us, good or bad.
Starting over, Shannon

Two Mommies-in-Waiting Share

My dream as a child was to be a wife and mother, and I loved babysitting. When I married, we made plans to begin "family life" right away. As each month passed without a pregnancy, I became more confused and discouraged and my prayers became intense. I called my OB-GYN in hopes she could enlighten me about our problem getting pregnant. She said that after a year of trying to get pregnant without contraceptives, she would classify me as "infertile." Until then, I don't recall ever hearing that word. She told me to keep track of my ovulation cycles and gave me other helpful tips. Wow! What knowledge I learned that day. I even went out and bought my husband boxer shorts.

It took me quite a while to figure out the cycles of my body. I never realized my periods were so irregular. I was faithful at taking my temperature every morning and charting all the important information. Several months went by, and it became increasingly difficult to keep the romance and passion in the bedroom without feeling we were involved in some type of lab experiment. I wasn't enjoying our sexual relationship at all. My sole focus was getting pregnant. — Gay Lynne

I became concerned when I'd been off the pill for six months and my period hadn't started, but I felt seeing a doctor might mean I wasn't having enough faith and trusting God. I was letting man fix my problem instead of God. But I felt God's assurance that he gave doctors the professional gift to help me and it was OK. I still was hoping to get pregnant without taking drastic measures. My gynecologist prescribed progesterone and Clomid to start ovulation, but I was surprised he didn't take any tests. After a year I changed doctors, but I didn't go to a specialist yet. The new doctor diagnosed PCOS. He ordered an ultrasound and ran tests which revealed I had one ovary twice the size of the other. A tubal dye study showed my eggs were maturing but not releasing. Insulin helps get the egg out of the tube, so he determined my insulin hormone wasn't doing its job and causing the enlarged ovary. He started me on a drug to get the insulin working properly, and I had a laparoscopy. Two weeks later, everything was back to normal, and in a few weeks I was pregnant. —Melissa

Janet's Mentoring Moment

For most couples, the first step in seeking medical intervention is seeing your gynecologist, preferably as a couple. The OB-GYN can do a laparoscopy, check for tubal blockage, determine hormone levels, and check the husband to determine if the problem is something minor in one or both of you that can be rectified without referral to a specialist. We often think of infertility as a woman's problem, but statistics show that "one third of infertility problems are attributed to the male partner, and according to the American Society for Reproductive Medicine, another third are related to both the man and woman."[1]

Another reason to start with your gynecologist is that he or she may solve the problem without an official "infertility" medical diagnosis, which might halt or limit insurance coverage. Check with your insurance company to see what your policy includes. Like Melissa, you might want to obtain a second opinion before heading to the infertility specialist.

Some couples bypass the gynecologist. Paula said, "When my husband and I decided the time was right to start a family and we hadn't gotten pregnant on our own during five years of marriage, we went straight to an infertility doctor."

Use the Peacekeeping Worksheet, page 257, to decide your next course of action. Every situation is unique. Follow God's lead after prayer, research, and discussion.

God's Love Letter to You

Dear_____ and _____,

Whoever obeys my command will come to no harm, and the wise heart will know the proper time and procedure. For there is a proper time and procedure for every matter, though your misery weighs heavily upon you (Eccles. 8:5–6, paraphrased).

Wisely yours, God

Couple's Prayer

Father, It's scary taking these first medical steps. We want to know if something is wrong, and yet we're praying everything is fine or easily fixed. Give us wisdom, Lord, as we venture into this unknown territory, a place we never wanted to go. We know you want the best for us, and we couldn't go on this journey without you. Thank you for always being there for us. Amen.

HOLISTIC MEDICINE AND DIET

*The medical side of infertility treatment is so planned
and controlled, you think that if you just eat the right things,
or do acupuncture, you can control the situation.*[2]
—Mary Nelson, in Heidi Schlumpf's, "Inconceivable"

HE MAKES THE WHOLE BODY FIT TOGETHER PERFECTLY. AS EACH PART DOES
ITS OWN SPECIAL WORK, IT HELPS THE OTHER PARTS GROW, SO THAT THE
WHOLE BODY IS HEALTHY AND GROWING AND FULL OF LOVE.
—Ephesians 4:16 NLT

Kim's Journal

Dear God,

I'm waiting a year before talking to my OB-GYN about my period not starting after going off "the pill." I've heard it sometimes takes several months before your cycle returns to normal. I should wait that long anyway before trying to get pregnant so the pill can clear out of my system. Besides, it's nearly impossible to get in to see my OB-GYN unless you're pregnant! It's just another stab that my life as a mother-to-be is pushed back because of all those lucky pregnant women who can see the doctor anytime they want.

In the meantime, I'm going to the acupuncturist three times a week. I've heard that acupuncture helps some women get pregnant, and it's a "natural" method without the use of hormones. So here I am, the person who faints at the side of blood getting pins poked into me, even on my scalp. The doctor wants me to eat all sorts of crazy foods to cleanse my body. One week it's all white food, the next it's orange foods. Crazy, but I'm doing it. I'm desperate.

Naturally yours, Kim

A Mommy- and Daddy-in-Waiting Share

Heidi Schlumpf wrote in her article "Inconceivable" about a couple who said they tried "everything":

> Mary and Sam Nelson of Denver [names have been changed] married in their late 30s and spent six years trying to have a child. They tried everything: acupuncture, diet, drugs, prayer, and eventually in vitro fertilization.

Not only were their attempts unsuccessful, but they raised difficult moral decisions and cost tens of thousands of dollars.[3]

Janet's Mentoring Moment

Shannon saw a holistic doctor, took herbs, and also did acupuncture. She said, "Acupuncture helped my body with the hormones and made me feel like I was doing something when a lot of this was out of my control. My body relaxed, and during a trial I saw the improvement in my egg growth and quality." A scientific review suggests that acupuncture might improve the odds of conceiving if done right before or after embryos are placed in the womb, but it hasn't been proven yet and is only theory. However, some fertility specialists say they are hopeful this simple treatment might ultimately prove to be a useful add-on to traditional methods.[4]

Nutritionally, Kim, Shannon, and I began reading labels, buying organic food, eating raw fruits and vegetables, and eliminating processed foods. We knew better eating habits probably wouldn't cure my breast cancer or necessarily result in pregnancy for the girls (although we were hopeful), but good food would certainly keep us healthier. It also gave us a sense of doing something to help our conditions.

"Want a Baby? Hold the Fries" was the title of an article reporting the results of research at the Harvard School of Public Health in Boston. The article stated, "The more trans fats a woman eats, the more likely she is to be infertile. . . . It's really a small amount of trans fatty acids that we observe having a significant effect on infertility."[5] Trans fats are found in fried foods, packaged snacks, commercial baked goods—anything with hydrogenated or partially hydrogenated oils listed as ingredients—so read labels.

Another study links caffeine with infertility. "If you're pregnant or want to have a baby, cut out caffeine or drink no more than one cup a day," says the director of nutrition for the Center for Science in the Public Interest. Their recommendation: one cup per day at most.[6] Kim went through withdrawal, cutting back to one cup of coffee a day, and Shannon only drank herbal tea.

You can't change your former diet, but you can start changing how you eat now. You might not get pregnant, but you'll be healthier and have more energy to pursue other avenues of becoming parents—and then you'll *really* need energy!

God's Love Letter to You

*Dear*_____ *and* _____ *,*

Why do you spend your money on junk food, your hard-earned cash on cotton candy? Listen to me, listen well: Eat only the best, fill yourself with only the finest. Pay attention, come close now, listen carefully to my life-giving, life-nourishing words. I'm making a lasting covenant commitment with you (Isa. 55:2–3 *The Message*).

The Great Physician, God

Couple's Prayer

Lord, Please motivate us to exercise, eat right, and do things as a couple to maintain healthy bodies and treat this great temple of life you gave us with the highest regard. We don't take our health and stamina for granted. Forgive us for any ways we've abused ourselves in the past, and help us work with you, the Great Physician, in fueling and maintaining our bodies according to your divine design. Amen.

WHAT'S NEXT?

I went through many, many infertility tests and procedures. Each time our doctor would say, "Everything looks perfect." —Gay Lynne

I PRAISE YOU BECAUSE I AM FEARFULLY AND WONDERFULLY MADE; YOUR
WORKS ARE WONDERFUL, I KNOW THAT FULL WELL.
—Psalm 139:14

Shannon's Journal

Dear God,

Well, it's been over a year of charting, learning about my cycle and my body . . . and I haven't gotten pregnant. When we started with the holistic doctor, I was so hopeful. The herbs were maintaining my cycles better than any birth control pills or surgery ever did. I thought we were on our way and this was our answer.

God, what should we do now? What's next? Should we see an infertility specialist? Maybe combine holistic and medical treatments? Three moms at my work have mentioned the same specialist. I wonder if that's a sign that he's the one to go to. One said she was pregnant within three months of seeing him. That sounds so wonderful. She also told me about tests she did, and some I haven't done yet.

Maybe it's time to read books about infertility. I never thought at twenty-seven I'd need to look at a book on infertility. What a word. The definition assumes something's wrong . . . yet you, Lord, say I'm perfect, complete, whole, and beautiful. I like the term "fertility specialist" because that's what I want him or her to make me . . . fertile.

God, help me as I research and read books and consider a fertility specialist. Remind me of your words, your hope, your love.

At a crossroads, Shannon

A Mommy-in-Waiting Shares

When we were first married, we talked of our desire for children but felt it was wise to wait a year before trying so we could enjoy each other and adjust to married life. A year and a half after our "I do's," at the age of thirty-six, we were ecstatic to discover we were pregnant. We had used a high-tech fertility monitor so as not to miss any opportunities. I was so excited for our first obstetrician appointment. Twins run in the family, so my doctor did an ultrasound. She questioned whether we had our dates right, and suggested we come back in two weeks to reassess the situation.

We prayed and prayed, convincing ourselves everything would be fine at our next visit. However, the doctor informed us it wasn't a viable pregnancy. The egg had not developed. Our hearts were broken.

When we tried again, we were pleasantly surprised to get pregnant after only two months, but five days after seeing the baby's heartbeat, I began spotting and we lost this baby, too. When genetic testing showed no abnormalities, our doctor sent us to a fertility specialist. If there was nothing wrong with the baby, perhaps there was something wrong with me. —Michele

Janet's Mentoring Moment

If the next step in your journey is referral to an infertility specialist, you have a decision to make. Some couples choose to forgo the specialist and pursue other avenues to parenthood such as adoption. Other couples take the plunge into the world of infertility treatment.

It's a pivotal decision. One spouse may want to go one direction, but the other is reluctant. Mary Nelson said, "Every time we got a phone call from the doctor, it was more bad news. It was heartbreaking. Sam was all set on adoption, but I was having a difficult time letting go of the dream."[7] Pray together to seek God's comfort and peace, and use Making Decisions and Developing a Family Plan, page 255, and the Peacekeeping Worksheet, page 257.

I know peace seems elusive, but God can help. No doctor, relative, or friend will have the right words or know the right thing to do, but God does. God knew you would face difficult times and decisions, so he gave you the Holy Spirit to indwell in your life and be your comforter. Talk to him. Pour out your heart and then receive the peace that passes all understanding.

God's Love Letter to You
Dear_____ and _____,
As a mother comforts her child, so will I comfort you (Isa. 66:13).
Your comforter, God

Couple's Prayer
Dear Father, We need comforting. It's a huge step from needing just a little help getting pregnant to needing science to get pregnant. We know we have options, but will they work? Should we try them? We're trying to remain hopeful. Let us feel the Holy Spirit's presence as we go into uncharted waters. We're seeking your direction and guidance. We feel you want us to be parents, but we don't know what step to take next in that process, so we wait on direction from you. Amen.

WHEN IS IT TIME FOR A SPECIALIST?

We visited the doctor and then we visited an infertility specialist. We spent so much time with our specialist that he began to feel like one of the family.[8] —Laura Christianson

WE'RE ADVISED BY THE EXPERTS. WE'RE SET.
—Isaiah 28:15 *The Message*

Kim's Journal

Dear God,
When I finally got an appointment to see my OB-GYN for my annual physical nearly a year after going off the pill, I sat in the lobby for what seemed like a lifetime. Of the twenty other women in the room, eighteen were pregnant and torturing me with their smiles and full bellies. As if this wasn't enough, the only reading material was parenting and pregnancy magazines! Mercifully, they finally called me in to see the doctor.

I told her my period hadn't started after going off the pill, and I wanted to have a baby. I explained I wasn't too worried at first, but as the months went by I became alarmed. The first thing she suggested was buying ovulation kits and testing at the same time every day for thirty days because it was possible to ovulate without having a period.

Filled with hope, I bought a bunch of kits on the way home and began testing. Thirty days went by, and nothing happened to that little stick to show any day was different from the next. What a letdown. Toby went back to the doctor with me, and she suggested trying Clomid for three cycles to help me ovulate. If I didn't get pregnant, it was doubtful more tries would help. She would give me a shot to "jumpstart" my period and provide a starting point to count the days to when I should be ovulating, then I'd take the Clomid and come back for a pregnancy test after a week. Well, God, not only was I not pregnant, but I still wasn't able to start my period after all that! What's wrong with me?

We went through this process for three months. With each "jumpstart" my heart was hopeful, and with each negative pregnancy test my heart ached. Then came the dreadful day she gave us the news: there was nothing more she could do and I needed to see a fertility specialist. I was heartbroken. She had said percentages were high for women getting pregnant on Clomid, so I was optimistic going into it. I remember thinking: *If this doesn't work, my chances of becoming a mother are slipping away.* Now we're really going to have to make an effort to become parents.

Brokenhearted, Kim

A Mommy-in-Waiting Shares

When we got married, my husband had a vasectomy reversed, and six months later we were pregnant. We were elated until at seventeen weeks I was miscarrying. Questions started going through my mind: *Did I lift something I shouldn't have?* To our surprise, an ultrasound showed we were pregnant with twin girls. One of the twins didn't make it, but the other twin was doing well, so I was hospitalized on strict bed rest. The next morning, my regular OB-GYN said there was nothing they could do. Nature would take its course, and since it was the weekend, a neonatal specialist would see me on Monday. Looking back, we should've demanded to see him right away. I lost both my perfect girls. The nurses wrapped one in a small blanket and put her in my arms. I was hysterical. Why have me hold my baby when I couldn't take her home?

I got pregnant again, but I lost this baby at four weeks' gestation. I was on an emotional rollercoaster: *What am I doing wrong?* Six months later, I was pregnant and went to a different OB-GYN but miscarried at eight weeks. Our HMO wouldn't approve seeing a specialist until I had three recorded dilation and curettage (D&C) procedures, and my second miscarriage had passed naturally.

A year later, I got pregnant and we were ecstatic. I was put on progesterone suppositories for the first three months, but the day after the ultrasound, the doctor called to say there was no heartbeat. I broke down. It wasn't fair! I want to be a mom. I deserve to have a baby. My husband and I would be excellent parents—give me a chance.

The next day I had a D&C. *Finally*, the insurance company approved seeing a specialist, who diagnosed that I had lost the twins because I had an incompetent cervix that opened up prematurely, thinking it was time to give birth. The specialist assured us he would help us bring a baby home. A year later when I got pregnant, we were excited but afraid of the unexpected. With the specialist, I had hope. We also had a different insurance, a PPO. I'll never go back to an HMO. —Marisa

Janet's Mentoring Moment

Marisa's story emphasizes the importance of taking ownership of your health and treatment and not relying solely on doctors. God gave us discernment and intuition that signals when something isn't right. We need to learn how to act on those signals and not remain at the mercy of the medical field. Marisa said, "We learned never to settle; always ask questions. If you don't like the answer, keep asking until you find your answer." The specialist did help Marisa have two successful pregnancies.

Doctors and specialists are skilled, intelligent people through whom God works and to whom he allots gifts and talents, but these humans can make mistakes or disappoint us. Don't be afraid to change doctors or get a second opinion if you don't feel you're getting the care you deserve or don't feel comfortable with the doctor. Your doctor should reflect your sense of urgency and desire for you to have a baby. When selecting a doctor or specialist:

- Ask family or friends for recommendations.
- Ask your OB-GYN who he or she recommends as a specialist and why.
- Check the Internet.
- Check what insurance covers.
- Visit an infertility support group and ask about doctors others are using.

- Pray and ask for God's wisdom in this important decision.
- Use the Peacekeeping Worksheet, page 257.

HMOs and some insurance companies put constraints on seeing a specialist, and some don't cover infertility. Know your policy well and be persistent in your request for the best treatment.

God's Love Letter to You

Dear_____ and _____,

Friends, guard Clear Thinking and Common Sense with your life; don't for a minute lose sight of them. They'll keep your soul alive and well, they'll keep you fit and attractive. You'll travel safely; you'll neither tire nor trip. You'll take afternoon naps without a worry, you'll enjoy a good night's sleep. No need to panic over alarms or surprises, or predictions that doomsday's just around the corner. Because I will be right there with you; I'll keep you safe and sound. (Prov. 3:21–26 *The Message,* paraphrased)

Your heavenly specialist, God

Couple's Prayer

Ah, God, Listen to our prayer, our cry—open your ears. Don't be callous; just look at these tears of ours. We're strangers here. We don't know our way. Amen. (Ps. 39:12 paraphrased)

MEETING THE SPECIALIST

We made an appointment with a well-known, local urologist specializing in male infertility. —Tiffany and Simon

SPECIAL MEETINGS—MEETINGS, MEETINGS, MEETINGS—
I CAN'T STAND ONE MORE! MEETINGS FOR THIS, MEETINGS FOR THAT.
I HATE THEM! YOU'VE WORN ME OUT!
—Isaiah 1:13-14 *The Message*

Shannon's Journal

Dear God,

I really enjoyed the experience with the holistic doctor and am hoping to find that same collaborative team effort approach with a specialist. Today, Dan and I met with the infamous Dr. Werlin, the fertility specialist I've heard so much about. He's very laid-back and has Rolling Stones music playing in his office. He fits with Dan's and my style. He had read our medical records before we arrived. How thorough! The office staff had set us up with an orientation and introduced us to the RESOLVE support organization before our first appointment.

In the office, I noticed bulletin boards full of cards, letters of thanks, and lots of baby pictures. I got hopeful seeing so many babies. Someone had even sewn a quilt with the names of children born that year. Everything told me he and his staff were special people, and the doctor said *he'd* call us personally to give test results. He joked with his staff and had an encouraging word for everyone. Many times throughout the visit and exam, he said to me, "You're perfect."

His encouragement meant a lot. Maybe he knew the stress I felt after years of trying to get pregnant and focusing on what's wrong with me, that I needed to be reminded how you see me, God . . . perfect, whole, complete. Thanks for the reminder. Thanks for giving us such a sensitive and thorough doctor. He and his staff seem to understand the importance of taking care of the whole person!

Hopefully, Shannon

A Mommy- and Daddy-in-Waiting Share

After years of trying to conceive without success, we *both* went to my gynecologist. He suggested testing Jim for infertility before starting anything with me. Jim did have a problem. This was heartbreaking news for both of us, and we suffered great pain and grief. We were referred to a specialist who offered a twenty-eight percent chance of conceiving a biological child through a relatively new medical procedure at that time. After praying about it and talking to our pastor, we didn't feel comfortable that was what God wanted us to do.

I became depressed and even bitter. So now what? Our dreams of becoming parents were seemingly dashed. We decided that since we couldn't have our own biological child, we should adopt since there were plenty of children out there needing a good home. —Jim and Brenda

Janet's Mentoring Moment

The infertility specialist's official title is *specialist in reproductive endocrinology and infertility*. Shannon likes to shorten Dr. Werlin's title to *fertility specialist*, focusing on becoming fertile, and Kim uses that term also. Other couples say *infertility specialist*. You'll see both terms used interchangeably in this book, but they're one and the same. Use whichever term feels most comfortable to you. A man usually consults with a urologist specializing in infertility.

Shannon said Dr. Werlin had been recommended by several friends, and she felt comfortable with him and his style. It's important to feel like you're going to the best doctor for your situation. Do your homework and research your choices before picking a specialist. Some doctors focus on specific aspects of infertility for men and women. If you know the source of your problem, go to the doctor who specializes in your condition and is knowledgeable in all the latest procedures. Use the Peacekeeping Worksheet, page 257, to prayerfully arrive at a specialist who is right for you. Use Making Decisions and Developing a Family Plan, page 255, to decide if you want to take his or her suggestions.

God's Love Letter to You

Dear_____ and _____,

Don't set people up as experts over your life, letting them tell you what to do. Save that authority for me, God; let me tell you what to do (Matt. 23:8 *The Message,* paraphrased).
Authoritatively, God

Couple's Prayer

Lord, Please help us choose the right specialist for our situation. You know the doctor who will fix things or provide options. This is a big step. Going to a fertility specialist opens the door for a diagnosis of infertility, and we're so uncomfortable with that word. But thank you for gifting men and women with knowledge and skills to help couples like us become parents. We especially want to find a doctor who appreciates our values and views. If further treatment isn't the direction we should be going, please make that clear to us. Amen.

Your Letter to God

No one enjoys going to the doctor. What have the appointments been like, and how has it felt telling your story, probably more than once? Tell God about starting down this journey of tests and procedures or your decision not to take that path. Be honest and share your heart, but don't overlook feeling expectant and hopeful.

Dear God,_____   Date:_____

_____

_____

_____

_____

Chapter Three

FACING THE DREADED DIAGNOSIS

GIVE ME THE BAD NEWS!
WHAT AM I DOING IN THE MEANTIME, LORD?
HOPING, THAT'S WHAT I'M DOING—HOPING.
AH, GOD, LISTEN TO MY PRAYER, MY CRY—OPEN YOUR EARS.
DON'T BE CALLOUS; JUST LOOK AT THESE TEARS OF MINE.
I'M A STRANGER HERE. I DON'T KNOW MY WAY.
Psalm 39:4, 7, 12 *The Message*

The Never-Ending Tests

The endless battery of poking and prodding tests produced no definitive diagnosis to our dilemma.[1] —Laura Christianson

I KNOW, MY GOD, THAT YOU TEST PEOPLE'S HEARTS. YOU ARE HAPPY WHEN PEOPLE DO WHAT IS RIGHT.
—1 Chronicles 29:17 NCV

Kim's Journal

Dear God,

The fertility specialist wants to put us through tests before weighing our options. Toby is having his sperm tested, and today I had a hysteropingogram (HSG) where they shot dye into my cervix through a very long tube and x-rayed where the dye traveled. It was a little uncomfortable, but I was praying this would give us some answers.

The dye lit up my fallopian tubes and ovaries so they could see if there were any blockages or problems. They told me that many women actually get pregnant after this procedure because the tube stretches everything and sometimes allows sperm to travel easier. So I'm supposed to go home and "try for the best with my husband tonight."

> Please, God, let this be the night! Let us be one of the "many couples" who get pregnant after this test. I'm hopeful.
> *Hopefully yours, Kim*

A Mommy- and Daddy-in-Waiting Share

Our infertility journey began after trying to conceive for a year. We went to an OB-GYN and had a preliminary fertility workup. While Tiff's results came back normal, Simon's test results showed he had azoospermia (no sperm). Simon's further tests with a urologist specializing in infertility came back unremarkable. We scheduled a testicular biopsy to find out whether in vitro fertilization (IVF) would be a viable option. —Tiffany and Simon

Janet's Mentoring Moment

The medical testing process can seem overwhelming and frightening and the terminology foreign. Use the Glossary of Infertility Terms and Abbreviations, page 249, and the Internet to locate definitions of terms. Most fertility specialists, or reproductive endocrinologists, have a standard course of tests that the American Society for Reproductive Medicine's practice committee advises as part of a *fertility* evaluation. Going to a fertility specialist is daunting, but until he or she conducts these tests, you haven't been officially diagnosed as *infertile*. The preliminary tests may show a relatively minor condition that can be easily "fixed," and you're on your way to making babies.

When additional testing must be done, unless there's a known problem with either partner, both the wife *and* husband receive testing. For a man, that means a semen analysis. Poor semen quality accounts for an estimated thirty to forty percent of all fertility issues, but it's an embarrassing and anxiety-ridden test that can lead to other serious problems. Judith C. Daniluk writes in *The Infertility Survival Guide*, "Many fertility clinics prefer that the sample be collected on site rather than at home, which can be a bit embarrassing and can present a challenge for some men. . . . Many clinics also provide erotic magazines or movies, or allow you to bring in your own in order to make the collection a little easier."[2] Daniluk's book, while informative, isn't written from a Christian perspective, and she is describing pornography. In the Christian fiction book *Desperate Pastor's Wives* by Ginger Kolbaba and Christy Scannell, a pastor and his wife discuss the potential dangers of sperm collection:

Jennifer took the slip from her purse, "[The doctor] wants you to go for a sperm test."

"A sperm test? What—he thinks this is my problem? Well, I don't need any stupid sperm test to tell me how to conceive a child. Besides, do you know what they do at those places? The rooms are full of pornography—videos, magazines. I counseled a man in our church who said his addiction to pornography started when he went for a sperm test."

Jennifer thought for a moment. She'd seen something about that in the infertility online bulletin board that she read sometimes when she couldn't sleep. "I'm pretty sure you can ask for the room to be cleared of that stuff."

Sam sighed, "But still. Come on, Jen. I don't want to be doing that in some room without you there. It's embarrassing."[3]

If possible, collect the semen sample at home and follow instructions for bringing it in to the clinic. If you're going to produce the specimen at the clinic, go together as a couple and insist on removal of *all* pornographic materials. Pornography is a sin. In your efforts to get pregnant, nothing justifies sinning. If it's too late and you've already used pornographic measures, go together before the Lord, confess your sin, and ask for forgiveness and God's wisdom as you make further decisions in this process.

If this test has started or fed a pornography addiction, don't ignore it. Run, don't walk, to your pastor and ask for help. As you seek God's blessings on your efforts to become parents, maintain integrity and do what is right in God's eyes. Pray for discernment to discard anything suggested in books, at clinics, or by doctors that you know isn't pleasing to God.

Take ownership of your treatment and ask the purpose of tests and procedures and what the results will indicate. Be proactive and don't hesitate to ask about a test you've heard about and would like to try. You are part of the medical team.

God's Love Letter to You

Dear_____ and _____,

My children, don't lose sight of common sense and discernment. Hang on to them, for they will refresh your soul (Prov. 3:21–22 NLT, paraphrase).

Watching over you, God

Couple's Prayer

Lord, We want to honor you in all we do as we try to have a baby. Help us remain forthright and make decisions pleasing to you. Give us opportunities to explain to others and to those treating us why certain procedures are not appropriate. Give us a discerning heart. We need you, Lord. Infertility is a test of our relationship with you and with each other. Amen.

THE AGONIZING WAIT FOR TEST RESULTS

I've had three miscarriages in a year. We got the test results back from the genetics lab on our last baby, and she died with Down syndrome. The other pregnancies had different problems, so the doctors still are baffled. I'm going to a genetics counselor. I fear it will lead to further tests. —Laurie

WAIT FOR THE LORD; BE STRONG AND TAKE HEART AND WAIT FOR THE LORD.

—Psalm 27:14

Shannon's Journal

Dear God,
The doctor did an ultrasound today. I always thought my uterus was small or deformed, and I was surprised it looked so big and normal! The doctor is testing both of us and will let us know the results as soon as he gets them. Oh Lord, the waiting is *so* hard. Sometimes, it feels like time is standing still as I'm going through this process. I'm waiting for my next cycle so I can do certain tests on certain days, all so I can wait for the results or take another test.

This is all I think and read about lately. I wish I had some answers, and it's hard waiting for them. I thought I'd come to the fertility doctor, he'd do a quick test to find out the problem, and I'd get pregnant. But we're still testing and dealing with the insurance company and what they're willing to cover. I'm excited to be moving forward, but why does it have to be at a snail's pace?
Impatiently waiting, Shannon

A Mommy-in-Waiting Shares

Waiting for the test results was so hard. Tiff's came back normal, but Simon's biopsy confirmed testicular failure and *zero* sperm production. We never expected to have problems conceiving once we started trying. We hadn't considered the possibility of not having biological children. This was quite a blow. Our emotions ranged from grief, sadness, anger, disbelief, and incomprehension much of the first few months. —Tiffany and Simon

Janet's Mentoring Moment

Waiting is never easy, especially when you're waiting for something you have no control over that could affect the rest of your life. At the same time, there's a sense of anticipation and hope. You walk a fine line to keep your sanity as you teeter between fear and expectation of the unknown.

Shannon said the devotional *In the Meantime: The Practice of Proactive Waiting* is "a very special book about what you do when you're not where you want to be in life. It's about the lessons we learn when we're in God's waiting room." Shannon wrote the following poem reflecting on the agonizing wait.

The Wait

Waiting, waiting, waiting—
Always waiting.
Waiting for a test, a procedure, a result,
An egg to grow.
All this waiting,
I can't tell if it's my friend or foe.
I get so anxious, so nervous, I fret.
Will this waiting end?
Will I have regrets?
All this time passes,
I watch many become moms,
and I wonder, "Is it my time yet?"
What will it look like when it is?
What will it feel like?
Will I know?
Will I glow?
More questions than answers.
I fret.
I feel caught between two worlds:
One of a mom,
One of a wife.
What will I be?
Can I be both?
My world would change so much.

Am I ready?
Will I ever be?
Will I doubt?
Will I fear?
Will I have nothing to say to listening ears?
Will I be selfish or giving?
Which side of me will appear?
Will I have a mommy voice?
A mother's instinct ringing in my ears?
Will I work, will I not?
What's my world to look like?
I can't tell,
It seems to be changing a lot.
Shopping's fun,
Spending time with friends is nice.
But they just pass the time
While I wait and wait.
What's going to be?
I can't see.
I feel like I'm losing me.
My figure, my skin, my sanity—
All fading.
Some days are great,
others aren't for the mentioning.
The sweats, the mood swings, the breakouts, the nausea, and ooooh the smells.
Did I mention the headaches?
Aches in my head I've never felt before;
It all seems too much.
Am I just complaining?
The me I knew is gone and I don't know who's come.
Lying flat on my back, "resting,"
Seems more like fretting.
I hate the wait.
Sleep, sleep, sleep.
It's my main activity lately.
The sun seems to go down so fast,
and days go by as I wait and wait.
The biggest question I ask myself is "What's coming?"
Can you tell it's the waiting I'm hating?

God's Love Letter to You

Dear_____ and _____,
Wait passionately for me, don't leave the path (Ps. 37:34 *The Message,* paraphrased).
Keep waiting, God

Couple's Prayer

We pray to God—our life a prayer—and wait for what you'll say and do. Our life's on the line before you, God, our Lord, waiting and watching till morning, waiting and watching till morning, wait and watch, for with God's arrival comes love, with God's arrival comes generous redemption. Amen. (Ps. 130:5–7 *The Message,* paraphrased)

THEY SAY WE'RE INFERTILE!

*We were wrestling with our combined infertility and
going through that state where you'll buy into almost any idea
to boost the chances of conception.* —Rachel L.

PILE YOUR TROUBLES ON GOD'S SHOULDERS
—HE'LL CARRY YOUR LOAD, HE'LL HELP YOU OUT.
—Psalm 55:22 *The Message*

Kim's Journal

Dear God,
Well, we didn't get pregnant the night of the HSG test. One more thing to get my hopes up only to be disappointed again. The fertility doctor said Toby's sperm counts and mobility are low. Everything appears normal for me, except I'm not ovulating. I can't have a baby, God, if I'm not ovulating. Why won't my period start? It looks like we're actually going to have to start infertility treatment. This wasn't how I thought we'd make a baby.
Disappointed, Kim

A Mommy-in-Waiting Shares

Having children was a "given" in my mind. I knew I was going to grow up, get married, and be a mom. The day the doctor told me I wouldn't be able to have children still is vivid in my mind, twenty-two years later. Anyone hearing "You're infertile" knows the head spinning, heart breaking pain of those words. I thought:

I'm twenty-seven years old, getting married in three months, how am I going to tell my fiancé Ray we can't have children? Numb as I was by the time I got home, I made the call giving Ray an option not to marry me. I'll never forget his reply: "I love you. I'm marrying you because I love you, not because we can or cannot have children." —Robin

Janet's Mentoring Moment

Until you hear those fateful words from the doctor—"You're infertile"—you cling to the thread of hope that your problems are easily fixable, and you'll soon be back on the road to making a baby. When the test results come back with a significant finding, your world starts spinning and shattering. Nothing prepares you for how you'll react.

Every doctor has his or her way of delivering the diagnosis. Some have you come in to the office, others call on the phone. They may be compassionate and understanding, or methodically focusing on the next step. However you hear the news, your plans are going to change.

Ask the doctor as many questions as you feel capable of hearing the answer to, and write the answers on Appointment Notes, page 259. When you've reached your intake threshold, make another appointment to discuss options. You're probably too emotional to make decisions. You need to hold each other and be held by God.

God's Love Letter to You

Dear_____ and _____,

I am a good God, a hiding place in tough times. I recognize and welcome anyone looking for help, no matter how desperate your trouble (Nah. 1:7–8 *The Message*, paraphrased).
Your hiding place, God

Couple's Prayer

Oh Father, You know our hurting hearts. This isn't the news we wanted to receive. *Infertile* . . . a word we never thought we'd hear. Lord, what do we do now? Which way should we go? How can we stand the thought of possibly not having our own children? Our only hope is in you, Lord. We cling to you and to each other. Amen.

Your Letter to God

How are you holding up through this process? What praises and pleas do you want to express to the Lord? Maybe you'll write a poem or a song to express your thoughts and emotions. Experience the healing of writing down your feelings.

Dear God,   *Date:*

_____

_____

_____

_____

_____

_____

_____

_____

_____

_____

_____

_____

_____

_____

_____

_____

_____

_____

_____

_____

Chapter Four

PARALYZING SHOCK

When I look back, I go into shock,
my body is racked with spasms.
—Job 21:6 *The Message*

A State of Shock

We left the doctor's office shell-shocked. Having a baby was going to be much more difficult and expensive than we thought.[1] —Cheryl Fields, "Infertility Tales," *Real Simple*

The doctors told us we would never have biological children. What a shock. That day marked the beginning of a long and difficult journey. —Tiffany and Simon

Stand in shock, heavens, at what you see! Throw up your hands in disbelief—
this can't be!
—Jeremiah 2:12 *The Message*

Shannon's Journal

Dear God,
We met with the fertility doctor today to get the test results, and I was shocked to hear my body was doing so well! I expected to hear all sorts of things wrong with me, but the doctor said all my blood tests were "normal."

I reminded him of my previous problems with endometriosis, but he didn't seem concerned. He did say there were some penetration issues with Dan's sperm, but he wasn't too worried about that either. In fact, he suggested starting out slowly, maybe with only Clomid! I was expecting something more, and I think I prefer a more aggressive approach. We've been married for seven years, and we haven't gotten pregnant. Something has to be wrong!
Shocked, Shannon

A Mommy-in-Waiting Shares

When I picked up the telephone, I couldn't have imagined the news my husband Ken had for me: his sperm count had come back zero! They were going to retest. Maybe a clogged testicular line, but surely not really a zero sperm count. But the moment he said it, I knew we wouldn't ever have a biological child. His mother felt guilty: What had she done to cause this? Ken was sad, but he was comforted that his condition was something he was born with versus something he caused.

Everyone was surprised and shocked but me: I merely was amazed. It hit me like a ton of bricks—how carefully God had planned that moment of my life. We actually felt lucky that we didn't have to endure multiple years of infertility. We got a big, fat no from day one! Some people thought I was in denial at the gravity of the situation. I realize it would be hard to believe had I not known the transformation God had planned for me. —Karen

Janet's Mentoring Moment

Every couple's infertility story mentions *shock* or a similar expression. Bad news is shocking and often unexpected. Even good news is unsettling when you're expecting the worst or the results don't make sense or provide a definitive answer. Our body reacts to shock—which can be defined as a sudden or violent disturbance of the mind, emotions, or sensibilities—with dry mouth, racing heart, sinking stomach, sweaty palms, numbness, flushed face, maybe fainting or sickness—a terrible feeling.

We can't live in a state of shock for long without the body completely shutting down. Mercifully, the shock phase passes and myriad reactions follow—denial, frantic research, anger, depression and, eventually, acceptance.

God's Love Letter to You

Dear_____ and _____,

I am holding you by your right hand—I, the Lord your God. And I say to you, "Do not be afraid. I am here to help you" (Isa. 41:13 NLT, paraphrased).
Your shock absorber, God

Couple's Prayer

God, We're sad and numb. We need comfort and reassurance that somehow we'll have a child. Help us process the news we've heard and accept the things we cannot change. We believe you're in this with us and you have a plan. Lord, help our love draw us closer together as we mourn this news. Let our situation grow our love and not divide us. We need you, Lord. \ can't get through this without you. Amen.

IT'S ALL SO CONFUSING!

What amazed me about this ordeal is that the medical professionals tell you so little about what's happening or what you can expect. I think more should be written on this matter so the whole undertaking isn't so scary. —Laurie

We had multiple visits to the doctor and heard medical explanations about my body that we only partially understood. —Michele

IT IS A LAND AS DARK AS MIDNIGHT, A LAND OF UTTER GLOOM WHERE CONFUSION REIGNS AND THE LIGHT IS AS DARK AS MIDNIGHT.
—Job 10:22 NLT

Shannon's Journal

Dear God,

OK, these words have been on my mind: I'm not sure what we're dealing with, but help me get through it. Lift me up, give me courage and strength. I'm scared; I'm afraid of losing it. I'm afraid of the unknown right now. As we're taking more aggressive measures, I've been reading books and accumulating information on the testing process . . . learning what test is for what and how to interpret the results . . . all about the terminology and options. I'm confused and feel overwhelmed. I find myself rereading sections I've already read and getting new stuff out of it each time. It's a foreign language. We're making choices and decisions we wouldn't have faced if we'd gotten pregnant naturally.

Confused, Shannon

A Mommy- and Daddy-in-Waiting Share

We were married fourteen years when we started trying to get pregnant, without any success. Tests showed Eric had an infertility issue, and blood tests revealed a slight case of cystic fibrosis making him sterile. The doctors told us we could *try* to achieve a biological pregnancy, but chances were slim to none. There also would be a chance of having a child with cystic fibrosis. We were devastated. Then the confusion started: Do we try to have a biological child when there's so little hope and the possibility of genetic problems? Do we go through IVF and possibly create more embryos than we can use? Do we adopt, or do we forget the dream of children?

Our intense prayer journey began. I wanted a biological child, but Eric was concerned about his genetics issue. We cried and prayed, cried and prayed. We both believe that when there isn't peace between us, the Lord isn't in the decision. Eric believed the Holy Spirit was saying he wasn't meant to have biological children. He couldn't dismiss his genetics. How could I, his wife, not respect and trust Eric's spiritual leading from the Lord? Devastated, I finally found peace with not having a biological child. —Eric and Kristina

Janet's Mentoring Moment

Anything unknown is scary. Doctors vacillate between vagueness and inundating you with confusing details, punctuated with technical, foreign-sounding terms. You're in new territory. It's natural to feel out of your comfort zone.

Most fertility doctors provide an inclusive information packet. Take your time studying it and focus only on areas that apply to your specific condition. The same advice goes for computer research. The Internet is a great resource, but you can drift into information overload.

Use the Glossary of Infertility Terms and Abbreviations, page 249, and write down questions you want to ask the doctor on Appointment Notes, page 259. Then take *Dear God, Why Can't I Have a Baby?* with you to doctors' appointments and record the answers to your questions and any new information or instructions you receive. If possible, go with your spouse, or ask someone to go with you to take notes. It's difficult to jot down information, listen with retention, and ask questions at the same time.

If the doctor's office calls at home and there's someone with you, ask that person to get on an extension phone to hear the conversation, too. Expect the unexpected. Be prepared—some things may throw you into shocked confusion. If the doctor or the office staff do anything unnerving, or you don't understand something, tell them. You may be helping the next patient. Obtain the answers to all your questions. If necessary, ask for another consultation appointment in the office or on the phone. If your doctor isn't patient, compassionate, and willing to give you time and explanations, consider another doctor.

The Peacekeeping Worksheet, page 257, will help with tough decisions. We'll talk more about this process in Chapter Seven, but for now, let God's promise in Psalm 32:8 bring you peace and comfort.

God's Love Letter to You

Dear _____ *and* _____ ,

I will guide you along the best pathway for your life. I will advise you and watch over you (Ps. 32:8 NLT).

Your guide, God

Couple's Prayer

Our Lord, In wonderment we pray. Should you, God, be told that we want to speak? Can we speak when we are confused? We cannot look at the sun, for it shines brightly in the sky when the wind clears away the clouds. Golden splendor comes from the mountain of God. You are clothed in dazzling splendor. We cannot imagine the power of the Almighty, yet you are so just and merciful that you do not oppress us. No wonder people everywhere fear you. People who are truly wise show you reverence. Amen. (Job 37:20–24 NLT, paraphrased)

I'M "ONE OF THEM"

It was hard for me to admit I was infertile. —Sharon

"YOU'RE ONE OF THEM." BUT PETER DENIED IT.
—Luke 22:58 *The Message*

Shannon's Journal

Dear God,

I feel like I'm always writing sad thoughts to you about disappointments. I intended my journal to be about pregnancy and being a woman. I wanted to write about happy things, not infertility! I wonder what the day will be like when I finally do get pregnant. It seems like I write in here once a year when a procedure doesn't work out. I'm so sad, God. Everything looked good this time around, and I was really hoping for good news. So many shots I can't keep count, a surgery . . . I'm miserable. It's overwhelming.

I now know this won't be easy. I want to move to a new place, new surroundings, new environment . . . something to distract me, something different than dealing with this. Maybe we could go to Europe and visit my sister Michelle. We need to gather money again for hormones, and this ICSI they talked about, assisted hatching, and all the retesting. It's so much to go through. I'm tempted to look into surrogacy and be done with it. Sometimes I wonder what I would do if this doesn't happen for us because being pregnant, being a mom, is what I want to do! It's all I think about.

Sadly, One of Them, Shannon

A Mommy-in-Waiting Shares

Here I was sobbing in public. I'd become like those poor women I'd been reading about online, who do nothing but think about having a child. I was standing in the drugstore checkout line holding the digital basal thermometer my doctor had ordered, so how could I not be obsessed? Every morning as I record my dysfunction, I'm reminded just how alone I am. Yes. I had become like those infertile Internet women. Many had gone into major debt. Some had lost jobs or friends. A few had lost husbands. I was determined not to go that route.

Dabbing at my eyes, I glanced around: Where was my husband? Moments before, he'd been standing quietly behind me watching me cry, again. I guess I'd finally run him away. He'd had enough of my emotional outbursts, my endless questions to God, my pain.

"Love," he said, using my pet name. My heart leapt and I kicked myself for being so irrational and melodramatic. Smiling, he handed me a small box of candy hearts. "I love you, Linda." —Linda Leigh Hargrove

Janet's Mentoring Moment

Verbalizing and acknowledging your treatments and procedures to get pregnant solidifies the reality that you've joined the ranks of a group you've been trying to avoid. Reaching that acceptance point is a good thing because now you can bond with couples in doctors' offices and support groups, and your commonalities can provide comfort that you're not alone on this journey.

It may take awhile to accept this new identity. Don't worry if you're not ready to be "one of them." When you do embrace this courageous group of couples committed to becoming mommies and daddies, you'll see there's a thread binding you together, even though your stories differ. You'll develop a new sense of compassion. Prior to your own struggles, you might have heard others' stories from a remote, impersonal, detached distance: *Poor things. I'm so grateful that isn't us.* Now it *is* you.

Consider the work God wants to do *in* and *through* this experience. God never promises to remove us from our struggles, but he does promise to change our perspective. Linda Leigh Hargrove concluded her Mommy-in-Waiting story this way: "I smiled. Tears of relief and joy flowed down my cheeks. My husband cared about me and, in a small way, he did understand. He was there. In that instant, I knew that just as my husband was standing before me, my God was there all the more. God truly understood my heart and the hearts of all childless women."

God's Love Letter to You

Dear_____ and_____,

Even to your old age and gray hairs, I am God who will sustain you. I have made you and I will carry you; I will sustain you and I will rescue you (Isa. 46:4, paraphrased).

Your rescuer, God

Couple's Prayer

Lord, You are holy and awesome, but how did you let this happen to us? We're numb, over-whelmed, sad, resentful, mad . . . it feels better to let it out. Lord, help us move to the next step of acceptance. Remove any desire to isolate ourselves from other infertile couples or our world. That would be such a waste of our hurt. There's a new group of couples entering our life; help us embrace them.

Give us courage to reach out to those needing a touch or a hug and let others know when we need that hug ourselves. Help us remain compassionate, understanding, and willing to lean on each other when our paths cross. Amen.

WE'RE IN THIS TOGETHER

Even if the tests had indicated one or the other of us was "to blame,"
Robert and I agreed we were in this together. If one of us was infertile,
we both were.[2] —Laura Christianson

THEY ARE JOINED FAST TO ONE ANOTHER;
THEY CLING TOGETHER AND CANNOT BE PARTED.
—Job 41:17

Kim's Journal

Dear God,

It's comforting at family gatherings when Toby and I have so much to talk about with Shannon and Dan, as we all go through our infertility tests and procedures. Our husbands know more about how the female reproductive system works than most people.

But sometimes I wonder if Toby wants a baby as badly as I do. He's hesitant about moving forward with the fertility specialist's recommendations because it feels contrived to him . . . like if you want us to have a baby, it will happen naturally. He's afraid pumping all those hormones into my body will affect my health later, especially since my mom had breast cancer. He thinks I'm not eating enough or I work out too much. I know he's just trying to help "fix it," but his suggestion that I might have something to do with this makes me angry.

I'm confident our marriage can survive parenthood, but can we survive infertility? God, I'm getting anxious and I'm turning to you. What should we do? I'm more willing than Toby to take the next suggested steps. I'm not ready to give up. God, please help us come to a place where we're both at peace with what we should do. I want to be a mommy. I want Toby to be a daddy.

A loving wife, Kim

A Mommy- and Daddy-in-Waiting Share

Since it was Mother's Day weekend, and we were sad that the two foster brothers we'd been caring for went to live with family, we took a trip to get away and clear our heads. The drive was so quiet. I wondered if we still wanted the same things. Returning the boys had drained our souls; I didn't know if we were even on the same page anymore. Through limited conversation, we decided to wait a while before attempting to foster again and determine what we truly wanted. The drive was beautiful; it felt like we were ten thousand miles away.

The weekend was just what we needed. We found each other again, back on that same familiar page. We came to terms with God and realized we wanted what God wanted. We were at peace with the boys leaving and our hurting hearts were better.

On our drive home, I said, "I don't want to wait any longer!" Donald said, smiling, "I don't either!" We were ready. We were now on God's timing, and he was finally ready for us to become parents. The next morning a baby boy was born, and three days later, straight from the hospital, our future son came home to live with us. Jeremiah 29:11 continues to give us as much comfort today as it did that weekend. —Cindy and Donald

A Mommy-in-Waiting Shares

When I dedicated my life to Christ, I knew this could be a wrinkle in our marriage. Suddenly, Ken wouldn't be first in my life as Jesus took first place. But in true Ken fashion, he was open to my personal growth. Over the next six years, Ken continually commented that he liked the changes he saw in me. I was serious about growing my relationship with God; Ken was serious about growing our relationship with each other. As long as I went to Home Depot and showed interest in things Ken liked, such as playing golf, Ken attended church with me. —Karen

Janet's Mentoring Moment

Infertility affects *both* husband and wife, regardless of which partner has the problem. In marriage, you become a union of one in God's sight: "yours" and "mine" merge into "ours" in every area of life. Ken and Karen understood the importance of staying involved in each other's worlds. You'll read later how infertility and loss drew Ken to the God his wife loved.

Cindy and Donald went away together to reconnect. Men and women react to circumstances differently: men fix, fight, or flight, and women express, engage, and experience. It's how God wired us, but misunderstanding of gender coping mechanisms can cause significant problems between husbands and wives.

A man commonly goes into his "cave" and emotionally tunes out as he tunes in to television, computer games, the office, work, reading, surfing, golf, sports—whatever takes his mind off the problem and wherever he doesn't have to talk about it. Women need to talk. A husband in his cave leaves his wife feeling rejected, alone, and thinking he doesn't want parenthood as much as she does. Kelly relates: "My husband's seemingly detached and unconcerned attitude didn't help my mental state. Only later did I learn he was in denial. I felt isolated and unloved as Zubair slaved away night and day to establish our new company."

Most men don't stay in their caves forever—they need to process issues in their own time and space and then they reengage. Wives can give them that space by finding another listening ear with a family member, best friend, or mentor.

Differences of opinion also may arise in how to achieve parenthood. Melissa said her husband had an it-will-happen-when-it-does attitude, while she wanted to take immediate action. A couples' support group helps. Shannon said in their support group Dan become more engaged and comfortable talking about their issues, and she could talk to other wives. We'll discuss support groups in Chapter Eleven.

God put the two of you together for a specific reason. Be patient, pray for each other, and remember God made you unique as man and woman, but you fit perfectly together in the union of marriage.

God's Love Letter to You

Dear_____ and _____ ,

I, God, made marriage. My Spirit inhabits even the smallest details of your marriage. And what do I want from your marriage? Children of God, that's what. So guard the spirit of marriage within you (Mal. 2:15 *The Message,* paraphrased).
Presiding over your marriage, God

Couple's Prayer

Lord, We're trying to learn to celebrate our differences and not judge each other for reacting differently. Help us remember we're both suffering and dealing in our own way with this crisis in our life and marriage. Grow us closer together and don't let anything pull us apart. Guide us with your wisdom and give us courage to face the future united as one with each other and with you in body, soul, and spirit. Amen.

Your Letter to God

Individually and as a couple, this might have been a tough chapter to read while you grapple with a future different from your plans and dreams. How are you coping with those unexpected changes? How is your marriage doing? Do you feel any clarity, or are you still in a state of confusion? Use this time to pour out your heart to God. Let him give you a vision and a hope for your future.

Dear God, _____ *Date:* _____

_____

_____

_____

_____

_____

_____

_____

Chapter Five

ASKING "WHAT IF?" AND "WHY ME?"

I REMEMBER GOD—AND SHAKE MY HEAD.
I BOW MY HEAD—THEN WRING MY HANDS.
I'M AWAKE ALL NIGHT—NOT A WINK OF SLEEP;
I CAN'T EVEN SAY WHAT'S BOTHERING ME.
I GO OVER THE DAYS ONE BY ONE,
I PONDER THE YEARS GONE BY.
—Psalm 77:3–5 *The Message*

What If?

There were so many "what ifs" and "how wills," but we knew our plans had long been out of our control, so we decided to wait and pray. —Danette

WHAT IF SOME DID NOT HAVE FAITH? WILL THEIR LACK OF FAITH NULLIFY GOD'S FAITH-FULNESS? NOT AT ALL!
—Romans 3:3–4

Shannon's Journal

Dear God,

I can't help wondering: What if we had started with a fertility specialist earlier or kept on trying to get pregnant after our first year of marriage? Would we have had better options and more time to figure things out? Or what if I had gone to the fertility doctor before the holistic doctor? Or what if I had combined the two methods and taken the herbs while doing fertility treatments? I know this kind of thinking isn't helping me, and we can't go back and change things now, but I can't help thinking what if it never happens? What would we do?

What-Ifing, Shannon

A Mommy-in-Waiting Shares

We tried *everything* we could: vitamins, supplements, timing schedules, and a new doctor. All initial tests came back within normal ranges. We slowly started pleading with God: Why not? Was it something we did? Was there something we hadn't done and should have? I can only imagine what the Spirit said for us when we didn't know what to pray, when I cried but couldn't formulate a plea. I clung to the biblical stories of Hannah and Sarah. My comfort was thinking that perhaps the plan for our child would be so great that it wasn't time for him or her to come into the picture. From there I moved to understanding why Sarah laughed. —Mel

Janet's Mentoring Moment

Appropriately, IF is the abbreviation for *infertility*. You wonder *if* things would have turned out differently with different choices in the past, and you wonder *if* a baby is in your future.

God provides protection against and spiritual weapons for fending off Satan's arrows that pierce your mind and heart with wounds of doubt, unrest, guilt, worry, shame, and sorrow. Daily praying the "armor of God" found in today's God's Love Letter to You helps cast out "what ifs." You will face each day with renewed courage and faith. You'll experience restlessness until you rest in God.

You can't change the past or control the future—but the *present* compels the *future*. Discard nagging doubts by listing every "what if" you can think of on the What If page that follows, and then put a big X over the page. Let this exercise clear your mind and allow you to move on to what you *can* do to fulfill your dream of becoming parents.

God's Love Letter to You

Dear_____ and _____,

Both of you put on my full armor so that you can take your stand against the devil's schemes. For your struggle is not against flesh and blood, but against the rulers, against the authorities, against the powers of this dark world and against the spiritual forces of evil in the heavenly realms. Therefore put on the full armor of God, so that when the day of evil comes, you may be able to stand your ground, and after you both have done everything, to stand. Stand firm then, with the belt of truth buckled around your waist, with the breastplate of righteousness in place, and with your feet fitted with the readiness that comes from my gospel of peace. In addition to all this, take up the shield of faith, with which you can extinguish all the flaming arrows of the evil one. Take my helmet of salvation and the sword of the Spirit, which is my Word. And pray in the Spirit on all occasions with all kinds of prayers and requests. (Eph. 6:11–18, paraphrased)

Your what-if buster, God

Couple's Prayer

Gracious Lord, We're worrying and wondering if we should have done something different or started seeking help earlier. It hurts to have these thoughts and discussions, so please free our minds and hearts from the taunting and haunting of what might have been, and the worrying and fretting over what might happen in the future. We need your help to keep each other in the present and to give us courage in making the hard decisions going forward. Amen.

WHAT IF . . .

☒ _____

☒ _____

☒ _____

☒ _____

☒ _____

☒ _____

☒ _____

☒ _____

☒ _____

☒ _____

☒ _____

☒ _____

☒ _____

☒ _____

☒ _____

☒ _____

When you've finished—you can't think of any more "what ifs"—put a big X across the page and move on.

WHAT ABOUT OUR SCHEDULE AND PLANS?

The Master Plan I created as a young girl turned out extraordinarily different than what I had envisioned.[1] —Laura Christianson

JOB ANSWERED GOD: "I'M CONVINCED: YOU CAN DO ANYTHING AND EVERY-THING. NOTHING AND NO ONE CAN UPSET YOUR PLANS."
—Job 42:1–2 *The Message*

Kim's Journal

Dear God,

Obviously, things aren't going according to our plan. I want to quit my job and be a stay-at-home mom. That's what Toby and I have talked about, dreamed about, and planned for since the day we were married. We're both in agreement that we've saved enough money, and we've even worked out a budget to live on one income. What's going on? We're being responsible. Why aren't our plans your plans? Don't you see what wonderful parents we would make?

Now I don't know what to do. Should I quit work and focus on trying to get pregnant? Should I keep working while we go through the infertility treatments? Is that even possible? The treatments are costly, so it seems foolish to stop working. What should I do? I see a plan for our life and it includes babies! Please tell me that's your plan for us, too.

Still planning, Kim

A Mommy-in-Waiting Shares

When we went through premarital counseling with our singles' pastor, we created our family plan. We would have at least two biological children by the time I was twenty-five, then we'd begin the process of adopting more children. Our pastor also had us talk about what would happen if we couldn't have children without assistance. We established how we felt about assistive reproductive technologies (ARTs) and how that relates to God. We decided if our finances allowed for ARTs we'd go that route, but we wouldn't put ourselves into debt. —Mel

Janet's Mentoring Moment

There is nothing wrong with living by a plan and schedule. Our lives would be chaotic without organization. Often our plans work out and things tick along right on schedule, but we need to leave wiggle room in our life planner for the unexpected.

Shannon said she learned that you have to be flexible. Otherwise, you'll go crazy or be continually depressed and disappointed.

If you pray for God to direct your life, an interruption in *your* plans may be a "God intervention." Many of the couples sharing their stories look back and realize delays and schedule changes had to happen for *God's* perfect plan to unfold.

A decision to continue with infertility treatments will mean tests, procedures, and doctors' appointments to fit into your calendar. If you're considering adoption, call several adoption agencies to find out their procedures and requirements and consider how to schedule this process into your life. If you haven't established a family plan like Mel and her husband did, go to page 256 and work on one now.

The Bible tells us that "plans fail for lack of counsel, but with many advisers they succeed" (Prov. 15:22). Share with your doctor important dates such as finals at school, a deadline at work, or a planned vacation. Ask specifics about what's involved in the procedure you select so you can understand how to incorporate treatment into your life. Invite your doctor to give you wise counsel as to what activities you should eliminate and what tasks you can continue doing.

Submit every day to the Lord. Pray about your schedule and your plans, and embrace the psalmist's words as you awake each morning: "This is the day the Lord has made; let us rejoice and be glad in it" (Ps. 118:24). Use a pencil on your life calendar and keep the eraser handy.

God's Love Letter to You

Dear_____ and_____,

There's an opportune time to do things, a right time for everything on the earth: A right time for birth and another for death. A right time to plant and another to reap (Eccles. 3:1–2 The Message).
Your life-planner, God

Couple's Prayer

God, Please help us maintain flexibility and orchestrate our life around the plans you have for us. We want to be responsible and put our lives and schedules into your capable hands. Remind us that what looks bad today, you're planning to turn to good. Please provide stamina to endure any treatment or adoption schedules. Help us extend grace to each other, our doctors, and anyone trying to assist us in fulfilling our dream of parenthood. Amen.

WHY DOES EVERYBODY ELSE HAVE A BABY?

We both bore the pain of watching everyone in our family have children.
One dozen children had been born in our combined families during the
nine years of our infertility battle. —Sharon

DON'T COMPARE YOURSELF WITH OTHERS. EACH OF YOU MUST TAKE RESPON-
SIBILITY FOR DOING THE CREATIVE BEST YOU CAN WITH YOUR OWN LIFE.
—Galatians 6:4-5 *The Message*

Shannon's Journal

Dear God,

I wonder when it will be my turn. I watch our family having so many babies . . . seven to be exact. My sister Michelle and my sisters-in-law Janel and Julie are all on their second! We just moved into a new house in a family neighborhood on a cul-de-sac, and the house feels empty without a little one. I feel desperate, Lord. Why me? Why can't I have a baby?

I don't know what we should do next with our lives. Having babies is what we're supposed to be doing, but what do you do when you can't? I wonder if I ever will get pregnant and what it would feel like if I did.

Questioning and comparing, Shannon

Two Mommies-in-Waiting Share

Friends with babies surround me; I'm in a "sea of babies" at church. I'm going to baby shower after baby shower, and every week it seems I hear of another pregnant friend. I want to be happy for them, and I am, but it's a crushing reminder that it's not me.

One Sunday at church, I was holding a friend's baby who had fallen asleep in my arms. I physically ached for a baby of my own. My heart felt like it was going to burst feeling his precious little heartbeat, smelling his baby scent, and wanting so desperately to have my own. It hurt so bad. —Robin

Honestly, the feelings you deal with will overwhelm you at times. The most difficult part for me was constantly being happy for other people. Most of my friends were on their second and third child. Why is it that it feels like everyone, and I

mean *everyone*, is pregnant when you can't have a child? Don't get me wrong, I knew we would have a child but when, God, when? —Karen

Janet's Mentoring Moment

We become keenly cognizant of people in our same, or desired, circumstance. When you focus so intently on wanting a baby—many use the word *obsess*—suddenly it seems the whole world is pregnant, at least in your world. You may start avoiding public places, like malls or even church, where you might see babies or children or pregnant women.

"Unfair" feelings start erupting when others get pregnant, especially if their pregnancy happened easily, without even trying, unmarried, or worse yet—unwanted. You struggle to congratulate those who have succeeded where you haven't. You tussle with guilt over jealousy. How can you possibly live out the Bible's instructions in 1 Thessalonians 5:16 and 18 to be joyful always and give thanks in all circumstances? Lord, surely you didn't mean I should be thankful in a circumstance like infertility or watching others live my dream? But God does mean exactly that. Otherwise, bitterness will tear your heart apart, which might be how you feel right now—torn apart. Resentfulness doesn't bring you a baby, but it could break good relationships and your heart.

God's Love Letter to You today instructs you to be happy when others are successful because the Lord knows if you don't *rejoice*, you'll *regret*.

God's Love Letter to You

Dear_____ and_____,
Laugh with your happy friends when they're happy; share tears when they're down. Get along with each other; don't be stuck-up (Rom. 12:15–16 *The Message*).
The great equalizer, God

Couple's Prayer

Oh Lord, It seems everywhere we look couples are pregnant or cuddling their precious babies. Our hearts ache with empty arms, and we want what those happy parents have: a baby. In our desperation, we often avoid these fortunate couples because it's too painful. Help us, Lord, to be happy for them and not consumed with resentment. They deserve a blessing as much as we do. In our humanness we'll falter, but with your help, Jesus, we can sincerely smile and rejoice with others as we ask them to pray for us to be as blessed as they've been. Amen.

IS GOD PUNISHING US?

Examining ourselves before God, we asked him if there was sin in our lives that caused our infertility problems. We soon realized the miscarriages were not a chastisement for sin. —Alice

[JESUS] WENT ON TO OPEN THEIR UNDERSTANDING OF THE WORD OF GOD, SHOWING THEM HOW TO READ THEIR BIBLES THIS WAY. HE SAID, "YOU CAN SEE NOW HOW IT IS WRITTEN THAT THE MESSIAH SUFFERS, RISES FROM THE DEAD ON THE THIRD DAY, AND THEN A TOTAL LIFE-CHANGE THROUGH THE FORGIVENESS OF SINS IS PROCLAIMED IN HIS NAME TO ALL NATIONS."
—Luke 24:45–47 *The Message*

Kim's Journal

Dear God,
I often wonder if you're punishing me for something I did before becoming a Christian. I know you forgave me, but is infertility my penance? I can't think of any other reason you wouldn't let me be a mother . . . even though I know better . . . it still feels like punishment.
Feeling forsaken, Kim

Three Mommies-in-Waiting Share

During our first four and a half years of infertility, I struggled with depression. A lot of "Why me?" "Why can everyone else get pregnant and not me?" "What have I done wrong that I'm being punished for?" —Sarah

We produced few embryos and only two were usable. The day of implantation, we listened to the doctor telling the couple beside us that they had *great* embryos. He told *us* we would use what we had. The implantation left me anxious and worried. Less than a week later, the implantation failed. I spent three days sobbing in horrible emotional pain. I'd like to say I called on God and sought his strength and comfort, but I didn't. I felt like I was reaping the seed I'd sown when I was young. Out of fear, I had thrown away with both hands the ability to have children, and now I was suffering the consequences. —Melanie

More than anything, Jeff and I wanted to have children. What had we done wrong? Was there some sin in our lives or our families? Did the Lord know in his omniscience we wouldn't make good parents? —Danette

Janet's Mentoring Moment

A common misconception and untruth is that God is using infertility to punish you for past sins. Kim and Toby were new Christians when they married. Kim knew Jesus had forgiven her, but still she wondered if God was punishing her for past sexual sins. She had been on birth control pills for ten years, since age sixteen. She questioned if this was why her body wasn't "waking up" and ovulating after going off the pill. It might have been, but that was the result of *her* actions, not God's punishment.

My husband and I counseled Kim and Toby with the truth that when we ask Jesus into our hearts, admit our sins, and ask for forgiveness, he grants us grace fully and completely—wipes the sin-slate clean. God doesn't punish us, but choices and actions have consequences and repercussions. For example, in the following story, Gail's infertility was due to her body growing a protective membrane over her cervix after two abortions. Gail writes:

> Since the doctor recommended surgery, I had to tell my husband about the abortions. After hearing the details, my husband said if God closed my womb, then he would open it. I rejoiced, although I knew my husband wanted to be a father. Many years later, on the day after my fortieth birthday, I decided I was tired of dancing with fear. My husband really wanted children, so I put aside my selfish desires, fell on my face, and asked the Lord to open my womb.
>
> After eleven years of barrenness, within two months of that prayer, I was pregnant. At age forty-one, I gave birth to a son. At age forty-three, God gave us a daughter. Tears of unspeakable joy fill my eyes when tiny arms encircle my neck. With each hug, fragments of yesterday's torment vanish. With each kiss, healing balm fills my once broken heart. God restored everything taken by my past. He shined his light on the hidden treasures in my soul and gave me a future and a hope. He enveloped me in his love and washed me in his forgiveness. He anointed me with oil, draped me in royal robes, and placed a crown upon my head. I

am his daughter, a daughter of the King. Because of his mercy, I stand unashamed of my past. I pray for those caught in abortion's deadly trap.

God blessed the first couple, Adam and Eve, and told them, "Be fruitful and increase in number; fill the earth and subdue it" (Gen. 1:28). God planned for couples to live in a perfect, sin-free world and have babies. Then Adam and Eve interrupted God's plan by falling prey to Satan's ploy, and sin invaded paradise. We weren't supposed to incur sickness, sorrow, death, loss . . . infertility . . . miscarriage . . . and God suffers with us over the destruction of his original plan. Things never will be perfect again on earth, but God promises to bring grace and mercy to your challenges.

God's Love Letter to You

Dear_____ and_____,

What man or woman is there among you who, when your son asks for a loaf, will give him a stone? Or if he asks for a fish, you will not give him a snake, will you? If you then, being evil, know how to give good gifts to your children, how much more will I, your Father who is in heaven, give what is good to those who ask me (Matt. 7:7–11 NASB, paraphrased)!
Your loving and forgiving heavenly father, God

Couple's Prayer

Father, We've sinned and done things that hurt you and us. Please forgive us and help us not sin against you again. Thank you for your grace and mercy. We want to live our lives for you. If our infertility is the result of something we've done, or had done to us, we know you can make a way where there seems to be no way. You are a good and gracious God, and we thank you for being the Ruler in our lives and our heavenly Father. Thank you for loving us in spite of our imperfections. Amen.

NOTE: If this is the first time you prayed a prayer asking for God's forgiveness, and you're ready to become a Christ-follower by accepting Jesus into your heart and experience peace and forgiveness that passes all understanding, go to My New Beginning Prayer, page 245.

Your Letter to God

If you just committed, or recommitted, your life to God, talk with him here about how it feels to open the door of your heart for him to walk through and take up residence. If you're already a Christ-follower, how has that helped you put to rest the Whys and What Ifs?

Dear God, _____ *Date:* _____

_____

_____

_____

_____

_____

_____

_____

_____

_____

_____

_____

_____

_____

_____

_____

_____

_____

_____

_____

_____

Chapter Six

DEALING WITH PEOPLE'S REACTIONS

Words kill, words give life;
They're either poison or fruit—you choose.
—Proverbs 18:21 *The Message*

Telling the Family

Both of our families grieved for us when we found out about our infertility, and they supported us when we told them of the options available. —Tiffany and Simon

Nobody I know could possibly understand this pain, least of all my mother, because she had children! —Danette

Families stick together in all kinds of trouble.
—Proverbs 17:17 *The Message*

Shannon's Journal

Dear God,
I know my family is as devastated and disappointed as we are, and they're grieving with us. Some of them seem cautious about getting too excited about any of our options, but I've asked them to support us in whatever we choose to do. Others are ready for us to go for it and are excited.

Everything Dan and I do involves the whole family, so I plan on keeping them informed. I want them to know what we're trying and the results so they can pray for us and support us. I'm glad Dan feels the same way.

It does seem that whenever we get together with Kim and Toby at our parents' house, the conversation quickly turns to what tests we're each doing and how we're handling them. The guys talk about us getting pregnant as much as Kim and I do. It feels good talking with family going through the same thing, since Sean and Michelle aren't having any trouble having babies. That's harsh. I'm happy for them, but I wonder: Why, God? Why can't it be as easy for me?

Dan enjoys being around family, but family gatherings with children are a reminder to me of what we're missing out on.

Feeling left out, Shannon

A Mommy-in-Waiting Shares

When we got the news that Ken's sperm count was *zero*, meaning we'd never have our own biological child together, oddly enough I found myself comforting those around me: my sister who, of course, was newly pregnant; my younger sister, who had an eight-year-old daughter; and my parents, who took the news quite harshly.

Then there was Ken's newly married older brother whose wife got pregnant six months after their wedding. They called on speakerphone to give us the "great" news and brag, "We're having the first grandchild. We're taking the family name even though we know you love it and we're set on it (ha ha)." They really thought this was hysterical. It wasn't fair. —Karen

Janet's Mentoring Moment

As Shannon said, infertility affects the entire family. Your parents mourn their dream of being grandparents and watching their seed carry on through the next generation. There's no predicting how parents or siblings will react, but be open and honest if they say something hurtful. If they're supportive, thank them and acknowledge you understand this is hard for them, too.

As difficult as it may be for you to watch other family members having children, they could be just as uncomfortable around you. Gay Lynne's sister, Laura T., expresses the angst of the fertile sibling: "When it comes time to make the 'big announcement' to friends and family that you're expecting, it's usually a joyous time. But I was filled with dread at the thought of telling my sister Gay Lynne, who had gone through a long period of trying to conceive. I couldn't do it. It was difficult for me to comprehend how it felt not being able to get pregnant. It scared me to talk about it with her. I thought she would appreciate not discussing my pregnancy. My sister actually was in the process of finding peace with God, but I didn't know that at the time. I froze up with fear at having to face her with my 'good news.'"

Dave and I told Kim and Toby and Shannon and Dan we'd support and pray for their chosen journey toward parenthood. We assured them we would love an adopted grandchild. God had prepared us for that possibility when we married and welcomed each other's children as a gift to our hearts and family. When Sean and Michelle, my other "gift children," started having babies, I loved their children like they were mine by blood. I would do the same someday with Shannon's children and Dave with Kim's. We were Grammie and Grampa Dave to all our children's children, regardless of their origin.

Keep the lines of communication open with family members, and perhaps ideas in this chapter will provide useful tips for helping others determine whether they're being helpful or hurtful and ease the family awkwardness.

God's Love Letter to You

Dear_____ and_____,

Even if your father and mother abandon you, I the Lord will hold you close (Ps. 27:10 NLT, paraphrased).

Your Heavenly Father, God

Couple's Prayer

Father, Thank you that we can call you Father and know you will never leave us or forsake us. That knowledge comforts us as our family struggles with how to react to our infertility. Sometimes we're not even sure what response we want from them. Please be with family members as they try to support us and deal with their own grief or fear of being joyful around us.

Help us rejoice with those being blessed with parenthood and remind us that their children are our extended family. Don't let us ever withhold love, even in the midst of our own sorrow. We can do all things with your strength. Thank you for adopting us into your family—the Family of God. Amen.

PEOPLE SAY THE DARNEDEST THINGS!

Your loved ones will say all the wrong things. All of us who have gone through infertility agree on this point. —Laurie

I FOUND MYSELF IN TROUBLE AND WENT LOOKING FOR MY LORD; MY LIFE WAS
AN OPEN WOUND THAT WOULDN'T HEAL. WHEN FRIENDS SAID, "EVERYTHING
WILL TURN OUT ALL RIGHT," I DIDN'T BELIEVE A WORD THEY SAID.
—Psalm 77:2 *The Message*

Kim's Journal

Dear God,

People keep asking when we're going to start having children, as if I'm making a conscious decision not to! I try shrugging it off with an answer that we probably will "someday." Inside, I'm dying. Why are people so insensitive, and why do they feel it's OK to ask something so personal?

Everyone seems to think they're a doctor and they know the answer to my infertility. Then the advice . . . the number one thing everyone seems to say is, "Oh, you just need to relax." Or "You're young; you've got plenty of time." UGH! Help, God, they're killing me!

Wounded by words, Kim

A Mommy-in-Waiting Shares

My dear husband was the only one who really tried to comfort me in my grief. He didn't give me platitudes like so many others. He didn't pat me on the head and tell me, in so much "Christianese," to get over it. He held me and let me cry. Though, somehow, that wasn't enough. I still felt like no one understood . . . like no one truly cared enough to share my crushing pain. —Linda Leigh Hargrove

Janet's Mentoring Moment

Many infertile couples' stories mention how thoughtless and hurtful people's comments and advice can be, even in the church—*especially* in the church. "If someone comes to see me, he mouths empty platitudes" (Ps. 41:6a *The Message*). Debbie wrote, "I've experienced people in the church say some of the worst things ever to me with every good intention. Probably one of the most insensitive and painful is, 'Maybe God never meant for you to have children.'"

Often it doesn't stop with insensitive, intrusive questions or opinions about why you aren't having children. Other couples experienced hurtful comments regarding their method of becoming parents. Paula said, "Having consulted God first about our decision to do in vitro gave me consolation when thoughtless people would criticize us having triplets or say we didn't wait on the Lord long enough. I can confidently respond that children are a blessing from the Lord, and if it wasn't for the Lord, we wouldn't have them: 'Blessed are those whose quivers are full.' Even though it's hard and discouraging when people say those things, I know it isn't from God. I am confident."

You can be sure thoughtless, hurtful comments aren't from God. Here is how God instructs us to communicate with each other: "Kind words heal and help; cutting words wound and maim" (Prov. 15:4 *The Message*). And, "Well-spoken words bring satisfaction" (Prov. 12:14a *The Message*).

Most people don't mean to be hurtful: they innately want to say and do the right thing. They offer a cliché or something that minimizes your situation or feels patronizing because they're uncomfortable being around someone suffering. Try handing out The Top Fifteen Things Not to Say or Do, page 86, and Eight Ways to Encourage an Infertile Friend, page 88.

At times, you too may be the insensitive person saying the wrong thing. Just as we need forgiveness, God reminds us to "Forgive your brothers and sisters from your heart" (Matt. 18:35b NLT). And, "Above all else, guard your heart, for it is the wellspring of life" (Prov. 4:23).

God's Love Letter to You

Dear_____ and_____,

You must make allowance for each other's faults and forgive the person who offends you. Remember, I forgave you, so you must forgive others. And the most important piece of clothing you must wear is love. Love is what binds us all together in perfect harmony. And let the peace that comes from my Son, Jesus Christ, rule in your hearts. For as members of one body you are all called to live in peace. And always be thankful (Col. 3:13–15 NLT, paraphrased).

Peacefully, God

Couple's Prayer

Lord, You know the things people say that cut to the core. It makes us angry, and often we want to lash back or avoid them completely. Help us respond in love and not receive into our hearts anything not spoken in love. And, Lord, please guard our own mouths when we're tempted to say the wrong thing at the wrong time. Help us forgive those who hurt us as you have forgiven us. Amen.

THE TOP FIFTEEN THINGS NOT TO SAY OR DO

I believe in the front of every church directory there should be a list of things that you shouldn't say to people during times of grief, just like emergency preparedness in the front of the phone book. —Debbie

Make copies of this list to hand out to friends and family. Add one of your own for #15.

THE TOP FIFTEEN THINGS *NOT* TO SAY OR DO AND *TO* SAY OR DO TO SOMEONE EXPERIENCING INFERTILIY	
WORRY WEIGHS A PERSON DOWN; AN ENCOURAGING WORD CHEERS A PERSON UP. —Proverbs 12:25 NLT	
DON'T...	**DO...**
1. Talk about people you know with infertility. Good or bad stories aren't helpful.	1. Let me talk about my story and listen.
2. Tell me God is in control, has a plan, or knew it was going to happen.	2. Show me God's love.
3. Say "I'll pray for you" unless you mean it, or tell me to pray harder.	3. Pray for and with me.
4. Say "Call me if you need anything."	4. Do something for me.
5. Pity or patronize me.	5. Show compassion.
6. Avoid me. It makes me feel rejected, different.	6. Keep normal contact with me.
7. Take your cue from me as to how comfortable I am talking about it.	7. Act like nothing is happening, minimize my situation, or compare me with someone else.
8. Tell others, unless you have asked permission.	8. Honor my privacy.
9. Offer unsolicited advice or suggestions.	9. Support my choices.
10. Be resentful of how my infertility affects you.	10. Remember, this is about me.
11. Forget about me after the initial flurry of the diagnosis. This could be a long haul; I need you.	11. Let me grieve and that takes time. Stick with me.
12. Say you "understand" how I feel. If you haven't experienced infertility, you don't understand.	12. Listen without trying to "fix" it or make comments.
13. Ask me personal questions or give advice or suggestions.	13. Curtail curiosity.
14. Assume it's a "female" problem.	14. Understand this is personal.
15.	15.

SUGGESTED RESPONSES
WE WILL SPEAK THE TRUTH IN LOVE.
—Ephesians 4:15 NLT

Following are frequent unwelcome comments and suggested responses. Non-satirical humor often defuses uncomfortable situations. Your goal isn't to offend or embarrass the person. The responses shouldn't be said sarcastically, defensively, or angrily. Use this as an opportunity to be a good witness.

1. *"When are you two going to start a family?"*
   Response: What makes you think we're not trying?

2. *"You just need to relax, take it easy, rest more, or take a vacation."*
   Response: Then I might have two problems—no baby and no job!

3. *"You aren't getting any younger!"*
   Response: Are you fishing for an invitation to my next birthday party?

4. *"You're young—you have plenty of time."*
   Response: Time is the one thing we have too much of now.

5. *"You should take_____."* (They name some food, herb, or drug.)
   Response: I'll check with my doctor about that.

6. *"You should try_____."* (They suggest some sexual position.)
   Response: You mean we're supposed to have *sex*?

7. *"We need grandchildren."*
   Response: We need to be parents first.

8. *"That happens all the time."* (A couple adopts and then gets pregnant.)
   Response: Actually, it doesn't. You just hear about it more when it does.

9. *"There must be some hidden sin in your life."*
   Response: Jesus forgave my sins when I became a Christian.

10. *"You aren't praying hard enough."*
    Response: Are you offering to pray for us?

11. *"If God wanted you to have children, you would."*
    Response: Ouch! *That* hurts.

12. *"You need to have sex more often or less often."*
    Response: That's pretty personal.

EIGHT WAYS TO ENCOURAGE AN INFERTILE FRIEND

Laura Christianson—a contributing Mommy-in-Waiting and
author of *The Adoption Decision*

1. **Love by listening.** Don't give advice or try to fix things. Just be there. Warm hugs are the best gift you can give.
2. **Learn about fertility treatment.** Infertility is a medical condition that often necessitates medical intervention. If your friend is undergoing treatment, learn about the procedures so you can better understand the physical and emotional symptoms she's experiencing.
3. **Do something normal together.** Invite her to lunch or a movie.
4. **Arrange a childfree visit.** Being around children may be difficult for your friend. If you have children, avoid talking excessively about your own pregnancy, childbirth experiences, or children.
5. **Cheer on adoption.** If your friend decides to adopt, show the same enthusiasm you would exhibit if she were physically pregnant.
6. **If you become pregnant, share the news in person, if possible.** Understand that your friend will experience a mixture of emotions—happiness for you and sadness for herself. Don't pressure her to attend a baby shower.
7. **Extend sympathy.** If she loses a baby to miscarriage or failed adoption, send a card, flowers, or a small gift in memory of the child.
8. **Pray.** If you are a person of faith, pray specifically—on a daily basis—for something related to her struggle. E-mail or text your friend, letting her know she's in your thoughts and prayers.

Your Letter to God

If God brings to mind someone you need to ask for forgiveness or forgive, write his or her name in your journal entry and pray for the right time and place. Forgiveness frees you from the burden of bitterness getting a foothold on your mind and in your heart. Give praise for encouragers.

Dear God,   Date:

_____

_____

Chapter Seven

PREPARING FOR WHAT COMES NEXT

With your very own hands you formed me;
now breathe your wisdom over me so I can understand you.
When they see me waiting, expecting your Word,
those who fear you will take heart and be glad.
I can see now, God, that your decisions are right;
your testing has taught me what's true and right.
Oh, love me—and right now!—hold me tight!
just the way you promised.
Now comfort me so I can live, really live;
your revelation is the tune I dance to.
—Psalm 119:73–77 *The Message*

What Are Our Options?

We began a discussion that would alter the course of our Master Plan; a discussion that hinged on one pivotal question: Do we want to be pregnant or do we want to be parents?[1]
—Laura Christianson

We humans keep brainstorming options and plans, but God's purpose prevails.
—Proverbs 19:21 *The Message*

Kim's Journal

Dear God,
The fertility doctor suggested our first option was *intrauterine insemination* (IUI)—artificial insemination—since our test results appear normal except I'm not ovulating, and Toby's sperm need help getting to my eggs. I convinced Toby I would be OK and we could afford it, and he agreed to go ahead. We set our boundaries at one round of IUI and we won't pursue IVF. If IUI is unsuccessful, God, we'll move on to adoption.

The doctor explained I'd receive hormones to stimulate ovulation. Toby would submit a sperm specimen, which they spin and clean and inseminate far up into my uterus at the time I should be ovulating. The sperm won't have to swim so far in what could be a "toxic environment." Hmm . . . I guess a uterus can be toxic to sperm. We watched a video to learn how to prepare and administer the shots Toby would give me at home. Toby practiced filling the syringe, tapping out the air bubbles, and giving the shot to a dummy.

Oh God, this all was so overwhelming! The syringe was *really* big. We watched the video twice. Toby was so nervous about getting it right. I'm wondering if we're going to be able to do this. Please help Toby be OK with giving me the shots, and please let IUI work for us!
Nervously, Kim

A Mommy-in-Waiting Shares

After we learned of Simon's sterility, I would've done almost anything to have kids. The fastest, easiest way—you name it, I was considering it. Our doctors, pastor, and closest friends repeatedly told us to take our time and not make a rash decision based purely on emotion. Although making a quick decision was the one thing I *did* want to do, I also knew we had to explore our options and pray and seek to understand God's will. Our options were: sperm donor (DI), traditional adoption, and embryo adoption (EA).

Simon said he would support whatever route we took. My mom and friends asked, "Why not DI?" It would halfway fulfill my desire of having biological children as quickly as possible. But I had doubts. If this was what God wanted, why was I uncomfortable? How would Simon really feel about it? That struggle led me to explore and confront: Why was it so important for me to have biological children? My only answer: It was what I expected after marriage. It would've been great having a child who looks like Simon and me with the good and bad traits of our personalities. DI wouldn't fulfill that dream.

While looking at our options, a church friend mentioned the Snowflakes embryo adoption program. The information we read was strongly appealing. I would experience pregnancy, but more importantly, it would allow us to bring a child into the world who otherwise might not have that chance. —Tiffany

Janet's Mentoring Moment

Today's couples have various options and avenues to parenthood. If medically assisted conception isn't possible, doctors often present "third party" reproductive options: another person provides sperm, eggs, frozen embryos, or a uterus as a surrogacy gestational carrier of an embryo. Robin and Ray had the opposite situation of Tiffany and Simon: Ray was fertile, but Robin was infertile, and one option was using an egg donor. Robin writes: "Being obsessed with the all-consuming thought of having children, we sought a medical miracle. After many blood draws, trips to the doctor, and wearing "the patch," it was concluded I would be a candidate for the egg donor program. Many friends volunteered their eggs, but we never could get a peace about moving in that direction."

Additional options are foster care, domestic or foreign adoption, which Robin and Ray chose. Tiffany and Simon chose embryo adoption through the Snowflakes Embryo Adoption & Donation Program which matches infertile couples from all over the country with couples who have excess frozen embryos. The adopted frozen embryos are thawed and implanted by an in vitro procedure, allowing the adopting couple to experience pregnancy. Success rates are the same as any in vitro procedure. For more information about the Snowflakes program, see National Contacts, page 253.

Nick and Fiona chose surrogacy after watching a TV special on *60 Minutes*. They said, "After several years of trying surrogacy, we finally had two wonderful twin boys, but we had quite a few leftover frozen embryos. We decided that instead of spending a huge amount of money, time, and possible heartache to try for more children, we should concentrate on the two miracles we had. Again on *60 Minutes*, we learned of the Snowflakes program needing embryo donors. We shipped our frozen embryos from New Zealand, where we live, to the Snowflakes facility in California. After much paperwork, they matched us with a wonderful couple, who tried once with no success, but the second time they had twins."

Rachel L. and her husband chose another viable option: remaining childless. She wrote "People probably think the only happy ending to infertility is one of two options: you get pregnant or adopt. I'd like to offer up another option, though certainly not final. I could live the rest of my days mourning the children I may never give birth to, or I can pick that third and readily available option, and be content with growing my spiritual family. As a non-parent, I have the luxury of extra time and resources I would have spent on my children that instead can be used to bring more people into our spiritual family: more sons, more daughters. A mother to all of them; yes, I am a mother after all. This is as valid a calling as raising a traditional family."

Tiffany found the book *The Infertility Companion*, put out by the Christian Medical Association, helpful in evaluating options from a Christian perspective. "This book is based on biblical truths and concepts as well as current medical knowledge," she said. Appreciate the advice given to Simon and Tiffany: take time to pray and not rush into what seems the easiest or fastest way to becoming parents. Praying brings God into the equation and allows you to weigh your options together as a couple until you both feel God's peace. Remember: a mother's love comes from the heart, not the ovaries.

God's Love Letter to You

Dear_____ and_____,
If you need wisdom, you should ask me for it. I am generous to everyone and will give you wisdom without criticizing you (James 1:5 NCV, paraphrased).
Providing wise counsel, God

Couple's Prayer

Lord, It's so difficult knowing what to do. Where should we spend our effort and money? We want a child, but we also want your blessing. There are options and choices we never thought we'd be considering. We know you have a plan for us. Please help us stay within that plan. Give us wisdom, discernment, and peace. Amen.

TIME TO MAKE A DECISION

Once we realized what we really wanted was kids, not necessarily a pregnancy, the adoption option made more sense. The alternative was more high-priced procedures with a low likelihood of success. We quickly made the decision to adopt. —Dan, Gay Lynne's husband

I PRAY THAT YOUR LOVE WILL KEEP ON GROWING AND THAT YOU WILL FULLY
KNOW AND UNDERSTAND HOW TO MAKE THE RIGHT CHOICES.
—Philippians 1:9–10 CEV

Kim's Journal

Dear God,
I have mixed emotions. I'm excited we've made a decision, and we're finally going to make a baby. I mean, how could we not get pregnant with artificial insemination? But God, I also have feelings of anticipation and fear. There's a high chance of multiple births—with all the

hormones, I could produce multiple eggs. And how will Toby do with the shots? Will he be OK giving them to me? Will I be able to handle getting a shot five days in a row? And God, what if after all this . . . we still don't get pregnant? What will we do next? I want desperately to be a mother. If I'm not going to be a mother, then what is my purpose in life?
Worrying and wondering, Kim

A Mommy- and Daddy-in-Waiting Share

We briefly considered foreign adoption and had started the initial paperwork, when we heard about the Snowflakes program through Dr. James Dobson's Focus on the Family radio program. Individually and together as a couple, we began praying and asked family and close friends to pray we made the right decision that was in the will of God. We both felt released by God to pursue embryo adoption through Snowflakes. We were matched with a family and underwent the frozen embryo transfer and became pregnant only to miscarry at eight weeks. We suffered pain and grief again, and bitterness started to creep back into our hearts. We prayed, along with our family and friends, about what to do next and decided to try EA again. The first transfer didn't work, but the second one did and the wonderful pregnancy gave us our son. —Jim and Brenda

A Mommy-in-Waiting Shares

The decision was already made for us when we committed in our family plan not to do ARTs if we couldn't afford it. Our plan helped us not go over-our-heads into debt when our budget couldn't handle the cost of ART. Infertility is cruel that way—our desire begins to color every option. It puts blinders on and gives permission to make choices we otherwise wouldn't have made. There's always a new procedure, a new protocol to make you feel if you don't grab this option, later on you'll regret it. —Mel

Janet's Mentoring Moment

The purpose of this book is not to persuade you or to influence your decisions. As you read the stories of fellow infertile sojourners, glean helpful insights and discard the rest. The Bible says, "Do not be shaped by this world; instead be changed within by a new way of thinking. Then you will be able to decide what God wants for you; you will know what is good and pleasing to him and what is perfect" (Rom. 12:2 NCV). If you want to know God's will, you need to think like God, and that comes through prayer—individually and together—and reading God's Word.

In making a decision, every couple must weigh the moral, emotional, spiritual, and financial acceptability of options. You had a master plan to get pregnant; if you haven't already, establish a plan for your infertility journey. Use the guidelines for Making Decisions and Developing a Family Plan, page 255, and the Peacekeeping Worksheet, page 257. Then you can begin charting your journey on the Infertility Journey Map, page 258.

My husband and I have learned that if we're not *both* at peace with a decision, we need to keep talking and praying. Often we'll pray and consider issues separately and discover we arrived at the same decision. In complete unity, we know to go forward. If we're still at odds, we don't try to change the other's mind because we consider the lack of unity as a sign from the Lord that we aren't ready to make the decision.

You might be wondering about "give and take" and "compromise." You'll encounter some meeting-of-the-minds where you'll come to an agreement, or maybe agree to disagree, but compromise means one or both of you isn't completely happy with the decision—maybe feeling pressured to cave in or give up on your dream. Take your time to arrive at a *mutually* satisfying, prayerful, peaceful conclusion: it's probably the one God was hoping you would make.

God's Love Letter to You

Dear_____ and_____,

"I will instruct you and teach you in the way you should go; I will counsel you with my loving eye on you" (Ps. 32:8).

Your decision advisor, God

Couple's Prayer

Lord, Thank you that we can place our options before you and pray over them, seeking your good and perfect will. Please give us wisdom to ask the right questions and do appropriate research to determine what best fits our beliefs and desires. Please help us make a choice that would be pleasing to you and give us peace. Amen.

HOW FAR WILL WE GO?

We agreed we wouldn't give up on our quest for a child, no matter what. —Sharon

CAN YOU FATHOM THE MYSTERIES OF GOD?
CAN YOU PROBE THE LIMITS OF THE ALMIGHTY?
—Job 11:7

Shannon's Journal

Dear God,

When Dr. Werlin talked about IUI, I was excited about the thought of trying things we couldn't do on our own! Nothing was happening with the holistic route, so we were getting aggressive. I wasn't thinking, poor us, we *have* to do this . . . I was like, yeah we *get* to try these extra things.

Now we've experienced four failed IUIs! I don't tolerate Clomid, so the doctor is talking about trying IUI again with injections. But I've been reading about different procedures that bypass our sperm penetration problem, and I'm going to propose we skip the next conservative steps and go straight to in vitro. I want to be even more aggressive and try something that has a better chance of working, and maybe they'll get more information about what's wrong. And how great that they'll insert already fertilized embryos! We'll have not only one chance but three or four. The doctor's nurse said since I'm only twenty-nine, I might get pregnant really fast! I like those odds.

I had a dream we were pregnant. I know we're going to have a baby . . . I'm ready to take this next step . . . I don't want to waste any more time . . . but Dan is talking and thinking through the moral issues. You know he's more of a processor than I am. Help me be patient and wait on Dan's timing . . . which may be your timing.

Dreaming, Shannon

A Mommy-in-Waiting Shares

My husband Zubair and I exhausted the standard course of infertility treatments, including fertility drugs and artificial insemination. Sitting in the office of Dr. Lawrence Werlin, a leader in reproductive medicine, we listened attentively as he described *preimplantation genetic diagnosis* (PGD), a testing tool that detects abnormalities in three-day-old embryos. It evaluates the possible cause of IVF failure in women of advanced maternal age. The chances of conceiving increase because they only implant predetermined viable embryos. Research indicated an IVF success rate of thirty-eight percent for a woman of my age; coupled with PGD the odds should increase, but we could expect to repeat this procedure three times before achieving pregnancy.

We decided against the procedure after investigating the possible adverse side effects, and the thought of enduring 250 hormone injections over the four-month course of treatment sent shivers up my spine. On our way home from Dr. Werlin's office, we stopped for a cup of coffee to soothe our souls. A woman approached our table and began chatting about her adorable children. "I can't begin to tell you how wonderful it is having children," she began. "My little ones are my greatest joy in life. Do whatever is necessary to have a family."

"Wow, how did you know?" Zubair marveled. "We're seeing a fertility specialist."

"I had to go through infertility treatment myself to conceive," the woman remarked. Giving a backwards glance as she strolled away, she added, "But it was worth it!"

Interpreting this encounter as a message from God, Zubair and I rushed back to the fertility medical center to tell Dr. Werlin about our change of heart. Days later, PGD test results revealed three healthy embryos for implantation and a confirmed pregnancy two weeks later. —Kelly

Janet's Mentoring Moment

God often speaks through your spouse. It was almost two years before Shannon's husband, Dan, worked through the issues he had with IVF. Ethical, moral, and personal beliefs will influence decisions; honor and respect each other's opinions and concerns. Forging ahead with something only one of you wants creates a wedge, and as prospective parents, you want a marriage united in purpose. Judith Daniluk, Ph.D. advises:

> Ethical and moral dilemmas are often difficult to articulate. Frequently they come out as a general sense of discomfort with a particular option, without a clear sense of where that discomfort is coming from. You may not know exactly why you're uncomfortable with a particular treatment option, but you just "don't feel right about it." It usually means you need to delve a little deeper to find the source of your discomfort. It may be fear of the unknown; it may be grief over being unable to produce a child; it may be that the option in question is against your cultural or religious beliefs; or it may be that some part of the procedure doesn't seem moral or ethical. Mentally walking through the procedure step by step is often the best way to identify and articulate the real source of your discomfort.[2]

Obtain more information and research regarding the option causing discomfort. Speak with a pastor and discuss your concerns, and let him or her advise how your faith regards these issues. If you consult a fertility counselor, select one who can give you a Christian perspective. You may revisit decisions and find yourselves entertaining procedures and methods that a year prior you wouldn't have considered. Stay flexible, but allow space for one or both of you to reach the point where enough is enough.

God's Love Letter to You

Dear_____ and _____,
Test everything that is said. Hold onto what is good (1 Thess. 5:21 NLT).
Your moral guide, God

Couple's Prayer

Lord, We want to do what is right in your eyes. Help us know your will and your way. Give us eyes to see and a discerning mind. We're considering things we never thought we would have to know about, not to mention do. We're on a mission to become parents . . . what does that look like from your perspective? We want to surrender our will to your will. Please give us strength and courage. Amen.

Your Letter to God

Talk to God about your options and decisions. Use this time to brainstorm with God the pros and cons of each one: things often seem clearer when you see them in writing.

Dear God,   Date:
_____
_____
_____
_____
_____
_____
_____
_____

Chapter Eight

STARTING TREATMENT

YOU'RE MY GOD; HAVE MERCY ON ME.
I COUNT ON YOU FROM MORNING TO NIGHT.
GIVE YOUR SERVANT A HAPPY LIFE;
I PUT MYSELF IN YOUR HANDS!
—Psalm 86:3–4 *The Message*

You Want Us to Do What?

The doctor explained that if I get past my third month, I would have my cervix stitched closed (cerclage) to prevent it from opening prematurely. I would be on bed rest and NO SEX. —Marisa

"PAY CLOSE ATTENTION NOW: I'M CREATING NEW HEAVENS AND A NEW EARTH. ALL THE EARLIER TROUBLES, CHAOS, AND PAIN ARE THINGS OF THE PAST, TO BE FORGOTTEN. LOOK AHEAD WITH JOY. ANTICIPATE WHAT I'M CREATING."
—Isaiah 65:17–18 *The Message*

Kim's Journal

Dear God,
When we thought we were finally ready, we got started with the IUI process. The doctor gave me a hormone shot to "kick start" my cycle, then on a specific day Toby was to start giving me shots for five days. The first shot was horrible! We were so nervous. I tensed up and he had a shaky hand. I ended up with a huge bruise.
Tensely, Kim

A Mommy-in-Waiting Shares

I spoke to our pastor's wife on several occasions about our infertility issues. During a sermon on stepping out in faith, our pastor felt in his spirit that a woman who wanted to have a baby was going to have one the next year. When he told his wife, she immediately thought of me as being *that* woman. I accepted this as confirmation we would have a baby. When our infertility doctor called and asked if we wanted to have one round of free IVF by participating in a drug study, I believed God was working out his promise, so we accepted.

I found it easier to give myself the necessary shots thinking we would have a baby soon. I went every few days to have an ultrasound to see if I had produced enough mature follicles to begin the next step of producing eggs. I also endured several days where blood was drawn periodically throughout the day to provide information for the drug study. One day, I had my blood drawn thirteen times! I had bruises up and down my arms. —Melanie

Janet's Mentoring Moment

Tensing up physically or emotionally causes more pain. You're thinking: How can I relax with a big needle coming at me or during an invasive procedure? Pray before every shot and procedure. Breathe in the Holy Spirit, your Comforter and Counselor, exhale out the toxins of fear and anxiety. Another relaxing technique is envisioning a calm and peaceful babbling brook, gorgeous sunset, or snowy mountain. Soft music and the sound of a water fountain also are soothing.

God's Love Letter to You

Dear_____ and_____,
I know your pain and will make you good as new. You'll get a fresh start, as if nothing had ever happened. And why? Because I am your very own God, I'll do what needs to be done for you (Zech. 10:6 *The Message*, paraphrased).
Feeling your pain, God

Couple's Prayer

Lord, We want a baby so badly, but they're asking us to do scary and painful things. We're not sure if we can do this, Lord . . . in fact, we can't do it without your help. Thank you for being available for us to call on in our time of sorrow and need. We're going to be talking to you a lot in the next few months. We can do all things through your Son, Jesus Christ, who gives us strength and endurance. Amen.

OUCH! IT HURTS!

*It was hard for me to admit I was infertile. It was even harder
to take the fertility drugs by injection and to suffer so much
physical and emotional pain.* —Sharon

GOD SAVES THOSE WHO SUFFER THROUGH THEIR SUFFERING;
HE GETS THEM TO LISTEN THROUGH THEIR PAIN.
—Job 36:14–15 NCV

Shannon's Journal

Dear God,

I felt like I was going crazy when I was on Clomid . . . I was a real nut case. The doctor didn't warn me about this, but my friends who had gone through it prepared me. Then you know the horrendous pain whenever they do anything to stimulate my ovaries . . . and each time it gets worse. The headaches and pressure . . . I know I have to get through it, so I focus on the fact that only I can do this . . . no one . . . not even Dan can do it for me.

And now that we've decided on IVF, the shots! I hate needles and I'm scared of the pain! Already my hips are black and blue and I have to have my blood drawn almost every day. I'm going to try icing the area before the shot. Oh, God, I hope icing helps . . . it seems like we'll be doing this forever. I'm not sure I can stand it. Please help me endure the pain.

Painfully, Shannon

A Mommy-in-Waiting Shares

How many, if any, of the three freshly implanted embryos would survive was an unknown. I had endured one month of daily hormone injections prior to implantation, with three more months to go. I sobbed for hours nearly every day while applying cold compresses to the injection site, a feverish, hardened mass. I railed against God for his seeming injustice: "Lord, why are you putting me through this torture? You know I've been terrified of shots since I was little! Will this painful treatment even be fruitful?"

The one bright ray of sunlight throughout these four long, difficult months was the daily visits from Ann, a fellow church member and nurse, who administered the injections. She was much more than a nurse: she was a counselor, friend, and prayer warrior. Her compassionate hugs and tender prayers lifted my spirit. Our conversations were therapeutic for my soul. Chatting with her about normal, everyday activities diverted my attention away from my own problem. Single-handedly, Ann carried me back from the brink of insanity. She was an angel sent by God to minister to his emotionally and spiritually wounded child. —Kelly

Janet's Mentoring Moment

If you're feeling emotionally, spiritually, and (now) physically wounded, I hope hearing the stories of those who have gone before you offers encouragement that you're not alone, and you're going to make it through this.

At first, Dan was apprehensive about giving Shannon shots, but soon it became a routine part of his day. It was strange to look in Kim's and Shannon's cupboards and see the shot paraphernalia, but it reminded me to pray for these couples and what they were willing to go through to have babies, my future grandchildren. It was a privilege to encourage and pray for them.

If your husband is having difficulty administering the shots, you can use a visiting nurse service, or perhaps your mother, aunts, sisters, or neighbors could assist. Shannon and Kim both said icing the area before and after the shot helps tremendously, and after a while, Shannon said the shots were "no big whoops."

While the wife endures most of the ongoing pain of fertility treatment, there are situations where the husband has to undergo a painful surgery or treatment, too. Pray together as a couple before every shot and procedure, asking God to comfort and relax you and provide endurance for the pain and inconvenience. Pray each experience draws you closer together as a couple. Read Scripture aloud to each other, and listen to God through his Word. He's there with you. Pray together every day and every step of the way. Pray for your doctors and technicians.

God's Love Letter to You

Dear_____ and_____,

What a gift life is to those who stay the course! You've heard, of course, of Job's staying power, and you know how I, God, brought it all together for him at the end. That's because I care, care right down to the last detail. And since you know that I care, let your language show it. Don't add words like "I swear to God" to your own words. Don't show your impatience by concocting oaths to hurry me up. . . . Are you hurting? Pray. Do you feel great? Sing. Are you sick? Call the church leaders together to pray and anoint you with oil in the name of the Master. Believing-prayer will heal you, and Jesus will put you on your feet. (James 5:11–15 *The Message,* paraphrased)

Your pain reliever, God

Couple's Prayer

Lord, Please give us courage and strength to endure the physical and emotional pain. Help us learn to comfort and soothe each other and remain relaxed and refreshed in the midst of these treatments. Amen.

WHO HAS TIME FOR BED REST?

At my eighth week, I started bleeding, and the doctor took me off work
for the remainder of my pregnancy. I made it past my third month,
had my cervix stitched up, and went on complete bed rest for the
remainder of my pregnancy. —Marisa

I KNOW THE LORD IS ALWAYS WITH ME. I WILL NOT BE SHAKEN,
FOR HE IS RIGHT BESIDE ME. NO WONDER MY HEART IS GLAD,
AND I REJOICE. MY BODY RESTS IN SAFETY.
—Psalm 16:8–9 NLT

Shannon's Journal

Dear God,

The doctor says I need to be on bed rest for the first twelve weeks after the embryo implantation—I shouldn't even go upstairs. That's a problem since our bedroom is upstairs, so Dan is moving our bed downstairs to the dining room. Guess it's a good thing we never got a dining room table.

I've quit work, and I'm willing to do this if that's what it takes. I guess it's what I signed up for when we started this process, even though I know it's going to be hard because you know how I like to be up and doing things. But I'm excited to be taking the next step toward having a baby.

I *loved* the feeling of the embryos being put in me. The doctor and Dan only wanted to use two, but I pushed for three, so three it is. I'm lying here praying for them each to attach and grow. Help me, Lord, to endure the boredom and not become impatient with just lying around. I hope people come to visit and don't forget me while I hibernate at home, waiting for you, God, to help us have a baby.

Dan and I do have different visions of bed rest, though. I envisioned five days of lying flat and he would bring me meals, hang out with me, and watch movies. He envisioned three days of surfing, hanging out with friends, playing video games, and then going back to work.

Restfully, Shannon

A Mommy-in-Waiting Shares

Our first go-round with IVF wasn't successful. My husband wanted to try IVF again right away, but I wasn't as sure. I agreed, but this time I went into it praying, "If it is your will, Lord . . ." So one month later, we tried again. The doctor said she had learned more about our situation, and we probably didn't have to put in as many embryos this time. But my husband didn't want to take any chances, so we used four embryos, and three were successful. We were having triplets! I carried our son and two daughters to thirty-five weeks after spending the last two and a half months of my pregnancy in the hospital on bed rest.

At home, I'd been wearing a monitor that checked their heartbeats, and I kept going to the hospital when it didn't register correctly. My doctor said this was causing me so much stress that I would do better in the hospital—which actually was wonderful! It was a nice facility, and they took great care of me. I probably carried the triplets longer because I was able to rest and have around-the-clock medical attention. When our babies were delivered, all three were breathing on their own and healthy enough to come home with me. —Paula

Janet's Mentoring Moment

When I interviewed Paula and asked how she survived bed rest, her eyes lit up and she exclaimed how much she loved it. I was surprised because most women dread the isolation and confinement, but when she explained that having her needs met by hospital professionals relieved her stress, it made sense.

While some women like Paula are hospitalized, many like Shannon do their bed rest time at home. These women often describe feeling "sentenced" to bed, with the loss of independence, boredom, and frustration. No one can empathize better with a woman "stuck on her back" than a formerly horizontal sister. Volunteer "Bed Rest Buddies" and similar mentoring and support programs have emerged through local and national organizations. Several are listed on National Contacts, page 252, and you might check what's available in your local area. The Internet offers many sites with ideas of what to do while resting and forums to meet new friends in the same situation. Here are several tips that bed-bound mommies-in-waiting offer:

- Make a distinction between day and night. Change out of your pajamas in the morning, brush your hair, make your bed (or hubby make it), and spend the day above the sheets.

- Shop online or from catalogs for baby furniture, toys, and clothes.
- Ask for help.
- Call the meals ministry at church or set up a meals calendar with friends and family.
- Ask your husband to lovingly fill in the gaps.

If this isn't your first baby, you'll need to make care arrangements for your other children. Relatives pitching in are great, but also consider hiring outside assistance. Don't think you can manage kids from your bed. You'll end up a nervous wreck and probably won't follow the doctor's orders to stay put. You've already invested so much, so budget for child care and help with household chores. This is the time to call in any IOUs. When others offer to help, don't shun their assistance. Make copies and pass out Bless You! Here's Where I Need Help, page 266. When you're up and around, you'll be able to help others, but for now, it's all about you.

In our fast-paced, production-oriented world, resting has evolved to be a luxury more than a necessity. The Bible refers often to resting and relaxing, and you've probably heard the phrase "resting in the Lord." God rested when he was creating the world, and now he and you are creating a baby, so rest even if you're not "sentenced" to bed rest. It's a perfect time to enjoy an extended quiet time with the Lord. Consider resting as a prescription to help your body physically, while you grow spiritually by reading your Bible and talking to God. You'll look back longingly at these times after the baby, or babies, arrive!

God's Love Letter to You

Dear_____ and_____,
Go about your business without fretting or worrying. Relax. When it's all over, you will be on your feet to receive your reward (Dan. 12:13 *The Message*).
Resting with you, God

Couple's Prayer

Lord, Fitting bed rest into our schedule is a challenge, but the doctor said we must. Help us receive this time as a blessing and follow the doctor's orders and recommendations just as we have in other areas of the treatment and procedures. Please bring our friends and relatives alongside to support us and provide endurance and stamina for however long this takes. Rest our minds, bodies, and souls. Thank you, Jesus. Amen.

Your Letter to God

Treatment is an eventful time in your life. Some things you would like to forget, and others you want to record for the future. Journal them all and then forget the bad and hang on to the good.

Dear God, _____ *Date:* _____

_____

_____

_____

_____

_____

_____

_____

_____

_____

_____

_____

_____

_____

_____

_____

_____

_____

_____

Chapter Nine

COPING WITH THE PRIVATE ISSUES

GOD WILL HELP YOU DEAL WITH WHATEVER HARD
THINGS COME UP WHEN THE TIME COMES.
—Matthew 6:34 *The Message*

It's All So Invasive!

At the dinner table one night at our parents' house, Dan and Toby were discussing their sperm counts and mobility, while Shannon and I were talking about our procedures and shots. Our personal lives were no longer private. It almost was comical, if it hadn't been such a focus of all our lives. —Kim

WE PRAY THAT YOU'LL HAVE THE STRENGTH TO STICK IT OUT OVER THE LONG HAUL—NOT THE GRIM STRENGTH OF GRITTING YOUR TEETH BUT THE GLORY-STRENGTH GOD GIVES. IT IS STRENGTH THAT ENDURES THE UNENDURABLE AND SPILLS OVER INTO JOY, THANKING THE FATHER WHO MAKES US STRONG ENOUGH TO TAKE PART IN EVERYTHING BRIGHT AND BEAUTIFUL THAT HE HAS FOR US.
—Colossians 1:11–12 *The Message*

Shannon's Journal

Dear God,

It's eye-opening to talk with other couples who have to stop treatment because they don't have enough eggs or the eggs aren't viable. It's scary to be at the end of fertility options. I know, God, that I'm fortunate there are still things we can do—albeit painful things. I at least have a chance.

I have hope when I see the amazing things you have done for other couples who have gotten pregnant. If you can do it for them, I'm willing to put in the effort and time and endure the pain and invasive procedures to see what you can do for us.

IVF is new and exciting to me. I welcome the treatments and have so much hope because more invasiveness means I'll learn more about my body, get more answers, be monitored more closely and, possibly, get pregnant for once.

Hangin' in, Shannon

A Mommy-in-Waiting Shares

My husband and I had been trying to have a baby for years when we finally decided to try fertility treatments. On my appointment days, I woke up at 4:30 a.m. to drive almost two hours to a fertility doctor. I was given pills, shots, and more pills and shots. I had three ultrasounds a week and experienced hot flashes and other side effects, along with the very important "scheduled sex"—usually twenty minutes after the last shot! I had a surgery to rule out endometriosis and dye shot through my tubes to make sure nothing was blocked.

Ten months later, the specialist informed us he had no explanation for why we weren't getting pregnant. My husband could produce children; I could conceive children. He said he had seen this in less than one percent of his cases. Our next option was IVF. We expressed concern about our schedules coordinating with his office schedule. He reassured us there would be no problem: my husband could drop off his specimen, and if I came within two hours, they could perform the procedure. The thought of getting pregnant without my husband present was the line in the sand. As well as having to prepare for multiple births, since we wouldn't do "reduction." —Tressia

Janet's Mentoring Moment

Much of infertility treatment is uncomfortable and embarrassing. Gone are dreams of making a baby from one enchanted evening. Romantic encounters have been reduced to cold, calculated medical science. Your private life has gone from intimate to invaded. You may start thinking: How much more of this can we take? Conception was supposed to be pleasurable and fun, and ours is painful and stressful.

Shannon said it helped to talk to other couples who had gone through similar medical processes. Some had endured six or seven cycles of IVF before having a child, and that knowledge prepared her for the journey she and Dan had started together. They had to keep their focus on the end destination—a baby.

If you're making a baby with medical assistance, thank God for doctors and researchers devoting their lives to helping you have options. If you reach the "line in the sand" moment when the process isn't worth the potential, it's time to move on without guilt or regret. Each couple has their own invasive threshold, and none should judge the decisions of any other.

God's Love Letter to You

Dear_____ and_____,

Your body is a unit, though it is made up of many parts; and though all its parts are many, they form one body. . . . And the parts that are unpresentable you treat with special modesty, while your presentable parts need no special treatment. But I, God, have combined the members of your body and have given greater honor to the parts that lacked it, so that there should be no division in your body, but all parts should have equal concern for each other. If one part suffers, every part suffers with it; if one part is honored, every part rejoices with it. (1 Cor. 12:12a, 23b-26, paraphrased)

Honoring your body, God

Couple's Prayer

Oh Father, We're opening up to outsiders the most private and intimate areas of our marriage. Help us maintain the perspective that we have a clinical problem, and we're simply seeking medical assistance as we would for any area of our lives. We still want to treasure our intimate times together, and we need you to help us keep everything in balance. Amen.

HOW WILL INFERTILITY AFFECT OUR MARRIAGE?

Joe and I had an unspoken agreement that we'd remain childless, yet I needed to do something about the ambiguity. The counselor listened to our dilemma and suggested the larger issue was our ability to communicate our hopes and desires to each other. As she worked with us over the next year, we began to uncover our feelings about parenthood. —Char

FOR THIS REASON A MAN WILL LEAVE HIS FATHER AND MOTHER AND BE UNITED TO HIS WIFE, AND THEY WILL BECOME ONE FLESH.
—Genesis 2:24

Kim's Journal

Dear God,

The second day of shots some blood appeared in the syringe when Toby withdrew the needle. He panicked. We were instructed that if he saw blood it meant he struck a blood vessel, and the hormone would enter my bloodstream, a potentially dangerous situation. He was on the verge of tears, fearing he had done something seriously wrong. It turned out to be just a little drop of blood on the surface of my skin that retracted into the needle.

He said he couldn't do this any more. He can't stand causing me pain or harm. He doesn't understand how they could give him this kind of responsibility. I've convinced him he can do it. We only have three more days to go. But, God, the damage is done. We're arguing over everything. The stress of the process and procedures, pay schedules, shots, and sperm retrieval weighs on us both.

I know Toby wants children, too, but I keep feeling I'm leading us down this path, and he's going along for the ride—like I want this more than he does. He loves me so much, and electively putting me in possible danger *really* upsets him.

We're both so stressed over the task ahead of us that at the end of the day, we're at each other's throats. The romance of trying to make a baby is gone completely. It feels more like a science experiment.

Stressfully, Kim

A Daddy-in-Waiting Shares

Marrying Gay Lynne was (and still is) the happiest day of my life. It was the culmination of a search for a lover and soul mate, and I felt simultaneously proud of the incredible gift of my wife and humble because God entrusted her to me.

Several months into our marriage, an uneasy stress began to build as we both "expected" pregnancy, only to be disappointed month after month. My wife didn't have the same joy in her life she had when we first married. I thought it was because she needed more in her life than just me. I wasn't meeting her needs.

After years of trying to have a baby, the physical intimacy we once enjoyed was replaced by the mechanics of a sexual transaction. The disappointments left me in a state of confusion and desperation, which led me to say I was "OK" if God intended for us to be without kids. This made a lot of sense to me, but Gay Lynne received it as cold and unfeeling, even though my intentions were good. The result was disastrous, as my wife became suicidal when the life she once envisioned and hoped for seemed a never-to-be-fulfilled dream. —Dan, Gay Lynne's husband

Janet's Mentoring Moments

Beginning or discontinuing a treatment or process or "trying" to get pregnant is an extremely volatile and scary time, with emotions and tempers on edge. If the wife is taking hormones, in Shannon's words, "She's probably acting crazy."

Shannon's husband, Dan, went to every doctor's appointment with her. If possible, attend medical appointments and procedures together, combining efforts toward a common goal. Plan date nights where you talk about things other than trying to have a baby.

Don't hesitate to consider counseling with a reputable Christian counselor who allows you each to express feelings and fears in a neutral environment. Char (from the opening quote) said, "I didn't want to talk with a counselor! Counselors were for people who had problems, and I didn't have problems! I agreed to go, though, when Joe found a counseling center at a local church."

Enlist people who will commit to pray for your marriage during this trying ordeal. Extend grace and be patient with each other. Don't let your marriage become a casualty of infertility.

God's Love Letter to You

Dear_____ and_____,

I have told you all this so that you may have peace in me. Here on earth you will have many trials and sorrows. But take heart [trust and faith] because I have overcome the world (John 16:33 NLT).

Your heavenly marriage counselor, Jesus Christ

Couple's Prayer

Lord, Please help us maintain peace and tranquility in our home and in our marriage during this stressful time. We don't want our marriage to be damaged from our desire to have a child. Help us come together as one in flesh and spirit. We love you and we love each other. Amen.

FEELING INADEQUATE

The emotional rollercoaster of feeling defective every time I went for treatments became just as heavy a burden as not being able to get pregnant, so we stopped all fertility treatments. —Tressia

The stress of infertility began creating a wedge in our relationship—I no longer felt adequate as the husband. —Dan, Gay Lynne's husband

I WAS UNSURE OF HOW TO GO ABOUT THIS, AND FELT TOTALLY INADEQUATE—I WAS SCARED TO DEATH, IF YOU WANT THE TRUTH OF IT.
—1 Corinthians 2:3 *The Message*

Kim's Journal

Dear God,

Toby and I went bowling with mutual friends before we were officially "dating." One couple had a three-year-old little girl, and as Toby watched me play with her, he thought I would make a great mother. After our engagement, he told me that was when he knew I was the woman he was looking for to be the mother of his children. He also mentioned a tradition in his big Italian family was for the firstborn son of the firstborn son to carry on his grandfather's name. Since Toby was the firstborn son, I agreed to continue the tradition.

Now each step we take into the "unnatural" process of trying to conceive a baby makes me feel less of a woman and wife to Toby.

Doubting myself, Kim

A Mommy-in-Waiting Shares

My miscarriage was physically, emotionally, and spiritually draining. I tried being strong. I knew chances for a miscarriage were increased due to my age of thirty-six, but I questioned my body's ability to function as a woman. I was anxious to try again. I didn't have a lot of time to wait. I just knew God was OK with our plan. After all, we felt strongly he wanted us to have a family. —Michele

Janet's Mentoring Moment

For whatever reason, one or both of you has a body not performing as "expected" and that's frustrating, but it doesn't make you less a woman or man. Having a child together isn't the ultimate purpose of your marriage. You married each other for better or worse, in sickness and in health, and now those vows are being tested, but with God's help, you'll ace the test.

Talk together about feelings of inadequacy, and affirm your love for each other. Focus on the joys in your marriage and the way God is working through you in other areas of life. Indulge in activities where you excel: What makes you feel good about yourself? If you're good at tennis or golf or cooking, play more tennis or golf or whip up some delicious dinners.

Maintain your outer and inner appearance by eating properly, exercising, and spending time in God's Word, focusing on verses that emphasize that you are a beautiful, or handsome, wonderful creation of God.

God's Love Letter to You

Dear_____ and_____,

Dress festively every morning. Don't skimp on colors and scarves. Relish your life with the spouse you love each and every day of your precarious life. Each day is my gift to you. It's all you get in exchange for the hard work of staying alive. Make the most of each one (Eccles. 9:8–9 *The Message*, paraphrased)!
Your sufficiency, God

Couple's Prayer

Lord, Sometimes we feel inadequate . . . like we're disappointing each other. Having a child isn't going like we wanted or expected, and we're fearful this could come between us. Lord, give us your confidence that we're made in your image, and you never make mistakes. Let our love for each other shine from the inside out, and remind us that your strength is adequate. Thank you, Lord. Amen.

OUR BODY CLOCK IS TICKING

After nine years of marriage, Joe and I agreed we would try to get pregnant. But had we waited too long? Had we put ourselves at risk for birth defects or other complications? Would I even get pregnant at thirty-nine?

—Char

WILL SARAH BEAR A CHILD AT THE AGE OF NINETY?
—GENESIS 17:17

Shannon's Journal

Dear God,
We've been married seven years and no baby. I'm still at a good childbearing age, but Dan is three years older, and he wants to have our family completed by the time he's forty. God, we've got to get this going! Please let IVF be the answer.
Counting the birthdays, Shannon

A Mommy-in-Waiting Shares

For two years my husband and I had been trying to conceive. In the meantime, my biological clock was steadily ticking. Married at age twenty-four, I had been eager to pursue a career after earning a civil engineering undergraduate degree and two additional graduate degrees. At the time, it seemed sensible to postpone starting a family. A dozen years later, I realized I was beyond prime childbearing age. It looked like medical intervention would be necessary. —Kelly

Janet's Mentoring Moment

As you read in Chapter Seven, Kelly did get pregnant with IVF. They successfully had a baby, and they went on to have three more children naturally. For various reasons, many couples today are waiting later in life to have children. Often Shannon was the youngest woman in their support groups, and sometimes she didn't feel people took her situation seriously because she had more years to try. But being young actually magnified her concern because she was at the prime age to get pregnant—but had no baby. Likewise, "You're not getting any younger" comments cut deeply into the heart of a woman who all too well knows the number of her years. Dads worry about age, too; they want to be able to roughhouse and play sports with their children.

Avoid judging someone else's situation or comparing with your own. Any woman or man who can't have a baby is going to ask God "Why?" regardless of age or circumstance.

Women of Faith speaker and author Sheila Walsh wanted to have a baby beyond prime childbearing age. When she told her doctor's nurse she was hoping to get pregnant, the nurse joked, "You'll be lucky. All your eggs are probably hard-boiled by now!" Shelia proudly laughs, "My hard-boiled egg is almost fourteen and taller than me."

God's Love Letter to You

Dear_____ and_____ ,

Abraham and Sarah were already old and well advanced in years, and Sarah was past the age of childbearing (Gen. 18:11). Sarah became pregnant and bore a son to Abraham in his old age, at the very time I, God, had promised him (Gen. 21:2, paraphrased).
I know your age, God

A Couple's Prayer

Father in heaven, Please hear our prayer. Our age might be working against us having a baby, and we're starting to feel panicked. Lord, you created us, and you know the inner-workings of our bodies. If it's possible, please assure us that we'll have a baby; if you're directing us to have a family in a different way, please open our hearts to accept that possibility. Our maturity would help us be great parents, and we have so much love to give. Thank you. Amen.

Your Letter to God

Marriage intimacy has gone from private to public. Spend intimate time with God telling him your concerns.

Dear God,   Date: _____

_____

_____

_____

_____

_____

_____

_____

_____

_____

_____

_____

_____

_____

_____

_____

Chapter Ten

GETTING NEEDED SUPPORT

ALL PRAISE TO THE GOD AND FATHER OF OUR MASTER, JESUS THE MESSIAH!
FATHER OF ALL MERCY! GOD OF ALL HEALING COUNSEL!
HE COMES ALONGSIDE US WHEN WE GO THROUGH HARD TIMES,
AND BEFORE YOU KNOW IT, HE BRINGS US ALONGSIDE SOMEONE ELSE
WHO IS GOING THROUGH HARD TIMES
SO THAT WE CAN BE THERE FOR THAT PERSON JUST AS GOD WAS THERE FOR US.
—2 Corinthians 1:3–4 *The Message*

Should You Join a Support Group?

Finally, there were others who understood what it's like to want kids and not be able to have them. It was good to fit into a group, even though it was a group of infertile people.
—Sharon

IF YOU THINK YOU KNOW IT ALL, YOU'RE A FOOL FOR SURE; REAL SURVIVORS LEARN
WISDOM FROM OTHERS.
—Proverbs 28:26 *The Message*

Shannon's Journal

Dear God,
I'm so glad Dr. Werlin recommended the RESOLVE support group. It's wonderful having a place to express myself. The group helps keep the fears and anxieties from overwhelming me and spilling over into other areas of my life. Now that I have a place to talk about everything and leave it there, I don't talk about it *all* the time. There's nothing like being around people going through your same experience. God, I feel heard, understood, and accepted. Dare I say *normal*?

Often I feel like Dan and I aren't on the same page. I now know that's common for men and women. The group really brought us together. I learned to accept what Dan was willing to do, and I trusted it would be enough and stopped pushing for more or for him to be at the same place I was at the same time.

I also get to hear Dan's perspective, and he hears other women who have similar experiences as mine with hormones and emotions. It feels more like a partnership rather than things just happening to me. They've given us great stress management techniques and suggestions for nurturing our relationship and handling other people's reactions.

Each couple has different problems, and the sharing gives me a better perspective on our situation and an eye-opener to all you can do. I see so many couples with the odds stacked against them having children. Great stories give me hope and encouragement. I'm learning different procedures to try and good questions to ask the doctor.

It feels like the group is walking through this journey together. Our load is lighter because we share it and don't try to shoulder everything ourselves. God, infertility is such a tremendous load to bear, and it's so confusing with the many difficult decisions. Infertility truly affects our hearts deep down and touches on our identity as women . . . mothers . . . nurturers . . . and men as husbands and providers. We need people who appreciate our journey. It's helpful being around couples who understand how we feel, not to mention the support of knowing we're not alone.

Our support group is essential. I really look forward to our group night. Please, God, help everyone in our group become a parent.

Needing support, Shannon

A Mommy-in-Waiting Shares

We started going to a bereavement support group at our local hospital. I am the oldest mommy-wanna-be in the room, and we're the only couple with three babies lost. But we all do have a common ground of losing our precious babies. —Laurie

Janet's Mentoring Moment

Infertility support groups are comprised of couples of all ages and walks of life, but the most important commonality in every group of infertile couples is the desire to have a child. One in six couples experience infertility, yet many say they feel alone, suffering in silence. Don't let that be you. Like the many couples sharing in this book, there are couples in your vicinity who understand your pain. Hospitals and fertility clinics usually provide support groups. Shannon mentioned RESOLVE, a reputable national infertility organization, but it isn't Christian-based, so also check for a support group at your church or a church in your area.

Along with the RESOLVE support group, Shannon and Dan attended the Empty Arms and Grief Support groups at Saddleback Church, which also has an

Adoptive Parents Support Group. We'll talk more about grief in Chapter Fourteen, but a grief support group is invaluable. Numerous infertility and grief Internet chat groups, Facebook groups, and blogs function as cyberspace support groups, but use discretion before disclosing personal information. Find more information on sources of support in the list of National Contacts, page 252.

Visit several support groups before settling on one that works for both of you. Keep the following precautions in mind when joining a group, whether online or in person.

You'll hear about other doctors. If you're happy with your doctor, be glad others are happy with theirs, too. If you're looking for a new doctor or a second opinion, this is a good place to locate a referral.

You'll hear about other couples' treatments and options. Every situation is unique, so discern whether what you hear about is applicable to your issues.

Celebrate with successful couples and cry with those who aren't. If you're successful, share your happiness with sensitivity to those still waiting. Some won't react the way you hoped. Also, be sensitive to your reactions to others' success.

Respect each other's privacy. Don't share stories outside the group unless the couple has given permission.

Beware that the interaction may be painful. It could be too much of a reminder of your loss or what you're missing.

A support group, in person or online, won't be a panacea, but every journey is more enjoyable and tolerable when you're on it with someone who knows the territory.

God's Love Letter to You

Dear_____ and_____,
Don't give up meeting together, as some are in the habit of doing, but encourage one another—and all the more as you see the Day approaching (Heb. 10:25, paraphrased).
Your constant supporter, God

Couple's Prayer

God, Please help us reach out to others who understand our plight. Everything is so personal, yet we know we could benefit from spending time with couples who share our struggle. Help us be givers and not just takers of understanding and compassion. Give us each someone we feel comfortable talking to, and maybe we'll form new friendships. Guide us to the group you know is best for us, or if it's your plan, provide us stamina and courage to start a group ourselves. Amen.

A CIRCLE OF FRIENDS

We were waiting at the hospital when we learned the devastating news: none of our ten adopted embryos survived the thawing process! We hadn't prepared for that outcome. Throughout the last couple of years, our friends, family, and small group at church had been praying for us. We were thankful for their support as we grieved our loss and tried to decide what to do next. —Julie

A FRIEND LOVES AT ALL TIMES.
—Proverbs 17:17

Shannon's Journal

Dear God,

I made some great friends in the RESOLVE support group. Some go to our doctor, and I see them in the waiting room. We exchanged numbers and feel like we can call each other whenever we need moral support or someone to laugh or cry with who understands how we feel without needing words.

I met Stephanie in the doctor's office, and we supported one another during our procedures. I couldn't have asked for a better friend. While I was on bed rest, she came over and brought me lunch and sent me encouragement cards in the mail.

Thank you, God, for these new friends and for all our friends supporting us. Even though they don't always get what we're dealing with . . . they still bring dinners and come to visit. It feels like you, God, reaching out to us and loving us through our friends. It's wonderful!

Friendly, Shannon

A Mommy- and Daddy-in-Waiting Share

We walked alongside two of our closest friends through their journey of infertility: one couple successfully had three children through IVF and one adopted from China. In talking with both couples and watching them interact with their children, we saw that adopting isn't much different than having biological children.

While there are certainly some differences, many of the challenges, joys, and frustrations of parenting remain the same. —Tiffany and Simon

Janet's Mentoring Moment

A circle of friends provides comfort, as well as information and camaraderie. When Tiffany and Simon struggled with their own infertility, they already had walked alongside friends on a similar journey. Observing these friends helped them become comfortable with adoption. They were blessed by reaching out to support friends.

God may use others to speak to you or give you ideas you hadn't previously heard of or considered. Throughout Shannon's journey, I often asked how she learned about a treatment or doctor. "From my friends" was her usual response.

The true test of friendship is being the kind of friend we want others to be to us. That means even in the midst of our own pain, we pray for and support whatever our friends are experiencing. The first step to healing is helping.

I hope you have a circle of friends accompanying you on this journey. If not, strike up a conversation in the doctor's waiting room, at church, or in a support group, and make new friends.

God's Love Letter to You

Dear_____ and_____ ,
This is my command: Love one another the way I loved you. This is the very best way to love. Put your life on the line for your friends. You are my friends when you do the things I command you (John 15:12–14 *The Message*).
Your loving friend, Jesus

Couple's Prayer

Jesus, You are our best friend, and we thank you for our earthly friends and the new friends you're bringing into our life through this infertility journey. Help us support others and let them know when we need support. Even people who don't have the same struggles we do still have struggles. Help us recognize their need for love and prayer. Thank you for being our friend. Amen.

A MENTOR HELPS

God has blessed me with opportunities to mentor and counsel women suffering from infertility. He has given me a story he uses to touch others. God has given me hope out of heartache, and that's worth everything. —Sauni

ONE GENERATION WILL COMMEND YOUR WORKS TO ANOTHER;
THEY WILL TELL OF YOUR MIGHTY ACTS.
—Psalm 145:4

Shannon's Journal

Dear God,

Thank you for the women willing to share with me the things that helped them in their infertility journey. I especially appreciate those who said, "Call me with any questions," and I did. It was comforting that someone else knew what I was going through and would take the time to answer my many questions. God, I hope someday I'll be able to help others as much as they've helped me. Please remind me to do so.

Gratefully, Shannon

A Mommy-in-Waiting Shares

Without a doubt, there are incredible things God has taught me through the struggles of infertility—things I wouldn't have known had I not gone through that experience. Since then, I've been through many other difficulties, and in each one I've learned things about Jesus that I didn't know. I've experienced His peace that makes no sense. He has proven over and over again His faithfulness. That's why I know He would have led us in victory through childlessness had that been His plan for us. That's the kind of God He is: not only does He give us His presence and peace, but He grows us through the experience. Then He allows us to use those experiences to minister to others going through the same thing. God has given me the privilege of walking with others on the road of infertility because of my own journey.[2] —Chris Adams, "My Struggle with Infertility"

Janet's Mentoring Moment

As I've done in this book, I often use my own, or someone else's, story to help others going through something similar. God doesn't give us character-building experiences solely for our own benefit. He wants us using the many ways we've seen him work in our life to encourage and mentor someone going through a similar experience. We use our been-there and done-that experiences God helped us through to assure another person he'll help her, too, and so will we.

When Carla Drew experienced a miscarriage, she reached out to another woman who also had experienced miscarriage. In "A Sisterhood of Suffering," Carla wrote, "Her understanding was seamless. She never said 'things happen for a reason.' She did tell me how long the crying would last and everything that follows a miscarriage. The crying slowed."

While pampering herself at a spa, Carla discovered seven women in the room recently had a miscarriage and were willing to talk about it. "I was surrounded by understanding strangers," she said. Later, when a friend had a miscarriage and called Carla, "I talked to her. I cried with her. I told her how long the crying would last, and then everything else that follows. Her crying slowed, and helping her helped me."[3]

You may think you can't reach out to someone until you're successful at becoming parents, but Sauni (in the opening quote) wasn't a mom, yet she was willing to mentor others in how she came to a place of peace. Chris Adams mentors infertile couples considering adoption, since adopting twin girls was the answer to their prayers for children.

Heidi Schlumpf, in her article, "Inconceivable," says of Emily Holtel-Hoag who suffered secondary infertility, "A trusted mentor challenged her to think more expansively about other ways to bring life into the world."[4]

Titus 2:1–5 is the foundation passage for my ministry, Woman to Woman Mentoring. I paraphrase those verses this way—teach what you've been taught so you can train others to teach what they've been taught. That's mentoring: sharing life's lessons with others. Gay Lynne says, "Little did I know what God was preparing my heart for and how he was going to use every hardship in my life to minister to others going through the same thing."

God's Love Letter to You

Dear_____ and_____,

I, God, am able to make all grace abound to you, so that in all things at all times, having all that you need, you will abound in every good work (2 Cor. 9:8, paraphrased).

Your mentor, God

Couple's Prayer

Heavenly mentor, We feel so needy. We don't want to impose on others, but this is an entirely new valley for us where we don't always know the language or the way out. Please bring people into our lives to share with us the wisdom you've given them. Help us remain humble and willing to listen and learn. And, Lord, regardless of the end of our story, remind us to pass on to others what you teach us in the midst of our trial. Amen.

Your Letter to God

If you have a support system, thank God for his provision. If not, how has God been talking to you in this chapter about cultivating one?

Dear God, _____ _Date:_ _____

_____

_____

_____

_____

_____

_____

_____

_____

_____

_____

_____

_____

_____

_____

_____

_____

Chapter Eleven

ENJOYING THE GOOD DAYS

On a good day,
enjoy yourself.
—Ecclesiastes 7:14 *The Message*

There Are Humorous Moments

Our infertility story is full of laughter, tears, and God's amazing grace. —Karen

A CHEERFUL HEART IS GOOD MEDICINE, BUT A CRUSHED SPIRIT DRIES UP THE BONES.
—Proverbs 17:22

Kim's Journal

Dear God,

To keep from going crazy with worry during those daily early morning doctor's office visits to get my shot or blood work done before going to work, I watched men coming in to deliver their "packages." Many were in business suits carrying a little brown paper bag; others were in work clothes. They looked so embarrassed and awkward—poor guys. I actually would have felt sorry for them except it was so funny watching them quickly sneak in and out. While it was humorous, I also appreciated that Toby had been one of those men willing to be uncomfortable and completely out of his element.

Smiling, Kim

A Mommy-in-Waiting Shares

There were a few hilarious moments which helped us make light of some very intimate aspects of our fertility treatment. My husband "collected" his sperm sample at home in the morning, and I delivered it to the laboratory. Our instructions were to keep the specimen warm and close to our body, so I put the cup between my legs while driving. Then I started laughing at how funny this looked.

When I got to the lab and presented the cup to the lab technician at the desk, she turned bright red and was so embarrassed she took me back into the lab before she would take my "package," even though the waiting room was empty! My husband and I had a good laugh. —Melissa

Janet's Mentoring Moment

Seeing the title of this Dear God section might conjure incredulous thoughts: *There's nothing humorous about being infertile. Janet just doesn't understand our pain.* I do appreciate the seriousness of infertility, but I think you'll agree there are some humorous times. You're not laughing off your problems or making light of them; you're just giving yourself permission to have a good day.

Your body relaxes when you smile. Plant a big smile on your face and try being tense or stressed. You can't do it. Many studies substantiate that laughing is healthy: it's good for healing and for the soul. If you have other children, they need to see you smile. Laugh with them and at their antics. In your desire to have *another* child, don't overlook the *precious blessings* that God already gave you. Rejoice in being their mommy and daddy.

Watch funny movies—avoid tragedies and dramas. Your life has enough drama without acquiring a fantasy burden. Cherish funny times—there will be some—that are often overlooked or minimized by the seriousness of the situation. Laughter helps keep everything in perspective.

The Bible assures you will laugh again: "The nights of crying your eyes out give way to days of laughter" (Ps. 30:5b *The Message*). Life is never *all* bad or *all* good: don't let the serious eclipse the humorous.

God's Love Letter to You

Dear_____and_____,
There is a time for everything, and a season for every activity under heaven. . . . A time to weep and a time to laugh, a time to mourn and a time to dance (Eccles. 3:1, 4).
The Author of laughter, God

Couple's Prayer

Lord, We've been serious for so long, and we haven't been smiling much lately. Help us indulge in laughter like we experienced before setting out on this journey. Please put joy back into our hearts as we focus on good times and not just on disappointments. Lighten our burdened shoulders and spirit. Give us eyes to see and a willingness to acknowledge funny moments in our day. Remind us to cherish the many blessings you've already given us. Amen.

RECEIVING LOTS OF LOVE

God provided fellowship in the form of men and women dedicated to loving us, many of whom had undergone similar trials.
—Tiffany and Simon

GIVE THANKS TO THE LORD, FOR HE IS GOOD; HIS LOVE ENDURES FOREVER.
—1 Chronicles 16:34

Shannon's Journal

Dear God,
I have many new ideas from friends willing to share their journey with me . . . even to helping me find Dr. Werlin. God, I am so grateful for my friends, the love of my family, and a doctor who is so kind and loving. I really appreciate that he personally calls us with information . . . that makes me feel so special . . . which I really need to feel right now because fertility issues have been such a blow to my self-esteem. Sometimes I don't feel strong and confident or normal, but I love my doctor always telling me "You're perfect."
Perfectly, Shannon

A Mommy- and Daddy-in-Waiting Share

The effects and process of coping with infertility wasn't new for us. We had witnessed many of our closest friends, who share our faith in God, going through it. However, infertility took on a new light once we were facing it. When we first learned about our situation, friends who had gone through similar journeys were there to cry and pray with us while they encouraged and listened. Both our families grieved and supported and loved us when we told them available options.
—Tiffany and Simon

Janet's Mentoring Moment

In Chapter Six, we discussed people saying hurtful and thoughtless things or deserting you, but many friends and family also rally around. These are the times to savor. Replace unpleasant thoughts with remembrances of those who showered you with love and understanding.

Someday, God will use you to shower lots of love on someone else on this journey, but for now, let others bless you. Hand out Bless You! Here's Where I Need Help, page 266, and soak in how wonderful it feels when God uses his people to show his love for you.

God's Love Letter to You

Dear_____ and_____ ,

I give you a new command to love one another. Just as I have loved you, so you must love one another (John 13:34, paraphrased).

Love always, God

Couple's Prayer

O God, You are our God, earnestly we seek you; our soul thirsts for you, our body longs for you, in a dry and weary land where there is no water. We have seen you in the sanctuary and beheld your power and your glory. Because your love is better than life, our lips will glorify you. We will praise you as long as we live, and in your name we will lift up our hands. Our soul will be satisfied as with the richest of foods; with singing lips our mouth will praise you. On our bed we remember you; we think of you through the watches of the night. Because you are our help, we sing in the shadow of your wings. Our soul clings to you; your right hand upholds us. Amen. (Ps. 63:1–8, paraphrased)

SOMEONE'S PRAYING

Prayer works on so many levels. —Karen

WE CONSTANTLY PRAY FOR YOU.
—2 Thessalonians 1:11

Kim's Journal

Dear God,

My parents have put Shannon and Dan and us on so many prayer chains and asked all their friends and small groups to pray. I know you're flooded with prayer requests. It's comforting that people we don't even know are lifting us up in prayer to you. How could we not become parents with so many people asking you on our behalf?

Praising, Kim

A Mommy-in-Waiting Shares

My older sister and another dear friend, both married for seven years, had been desperately trying to have children. These women became my first purposeful prayer assignment from God after taking a Precepts Bible study class. Miraculously, my vigilant praying for them coincided with the beginning of my own baby journey. I wanted these dear women to feel God in their lives the way I had been feeling him, so they would know they could get through anything. When you feel that for real, you truly want to scream it to the world.

I prayed, "Please God, let them know your comfort and your love." My favorite Bible verses are Jeremiah 29:11–13, "For I know the plans I have for you." So there I was, trying to conceive myself and praying earnestly over these other women. Miracle above all miracles, with IVF and lots of prayers, both women conceived and the pregnancies took! I was ecstatic. Thank you, God! —Karen

Janet's Mentoring Moment

While trying to get pregnant herself, Karen prayed for her sister and friend. Even when they were successful and she still wasn't, she rejoiced and praised God victoriously for the answer to her prayers for them. Karen prayerfully chose joy as God prepared her for her own infertility struggle. She personified the challenge to "Love your neighbor *as* yourself" (Matt. 22:39, emphasis added). If you struggle to be happy for someone who is pregnant when you're not, praying for her will change your heart.

Many infertile couples hesitate to share their infertility with others, but the more people you tell, the more potential prayer warriors. Be discreet, but be specific about where you need prayer.

God's Love Letter to You

Dear_____ and_____,
Rejoice in me, the Lord, always. I will say it again: Rejoice! Let your gentleness be evident to all. I, the Lord, am near. Do not be anxious about anything, but in everything, by prayer and petition, with thanksgiving, present your requests to me, God. And my peace, which transcends all understanding, will guard your hearts and your minds in Christ Jesus. Finally, brother and sister, whatever is true, whatever is noble, whatever is right, whatever is pure, whatever is lovely, whatever is admirable—if anything is excellent or praiseworthy—think about such things. (Phil. 4:4–8, paraphrased)
I am near, God

Couple's Prayer

Lord, Thank you for all of those we know, and those we don't know, who are praying for us. We feel cared for and special. Help us remember to pray for others even in the midst of our own difficult times. Amen.

TIME TO CELEBRATE!

I thought, "Oh, my God, my heart is starting to grow again. I can love again. There is going to be happiness in my life" [observing the ultrasound heartbeat of a new baby after loss of a child].[1] —Cheryl Albrecht, in Karen Springer, "Love, Loss—And Love"

WHEN ELIZABETH WAS FULL-TERM IN HER PREGNANCY, SHE BORE A SON. HER NEIGHBORS AND RELATIVES, SEEING THAT GOD HAD OVERWHELMED HER WITH MERCY, CELEBRATED WITH HER.
—LUKE 1:57–58 *The Message*

Shannon's Journal

Dear God,

Well, it was our turn this time around. We're pregnant!!!!!!!! The doctor called and all the staff screamed it into the phone. I cried hysterically with joy and felt so overwhelmed with all the emotions. That's probably why it took me until now to write you about it. Tonight it came to me I wanted to write everything down before I forget. It took several days for the shock to wear off. The last few days we've been wondering how many embryos will implant. We'll find out in the next few weeks. Tomorrow is our first sonogram; I never thought I'd get to say those words or even see a positive pregnancy test. We're so excited!

Celebrating, Shannon

A Mommy-in-Waiting Shares

Since my second miscarriage, I've been in and out of doctors' and specialists' offices. After what felt like a million tests, everything checked out fine. We started trying again and are now just over twelve weeks pregnant with baby number three, and so far everything is going well. I'm being closely monitored and still going through more tests.

We're approaching what would have been the due date for my last little lost one, and we think that might be a good day to make the announcement to friends about our new blessing. It could be a day of grieving, but we've decided to change our attitudes and celebrate instead. —Laurelle

Janet's Mentoring Moment

There can be celebratory moments beyond having a positive pregnancy test or the phone call that you've been selected by a birth mom. Those definitely are over-the-top, rip-roaring celebrations, but some celebrations require a choice: Your pregnancy test is negative, but your friend's is positive. You're not selected as adopting parents, but an orphan receives a loving home. The foster child leaves your family, but he or she reunites with his or her own family. God does change mourning to dancing when we change our perspective: despair to delight, deflation to elation, unhappiness to happiness, discouragement to encouragement, disappointment to enjoyment. Celebrating doesn't minimize the loss, but it does emphasize the cross.

God's Love Letter to You

Dear_____ and_____,
Rejoice! Celebrate all the good things that God, your God, has given you and your family (Deut. 26:11 *The Message*).
Rejoicing, God

Couple's Prayer

Oh Jesus, Don't let us ever miss an opportunity to celebrate the good things you bring into our lives. Remind us to celebrate anniversaries, birthdays, promotions, holidays . . . regardless of the trial we're enduring at the time. And help us never minimize the wonderful things you do for us *every* day and the sacrifice you made for us. Remind us to celebrate your birth and resurrection. In Jesus' name. Amen.

Your Letter to God

This is a good place and time to record the good days you've experienced, so when the hard days come, and they will, you can look back and remember all that God and others have done for you.

Dear God,_____ Date:_____
_____
_____

_____

_____

_____

_____

_____

_____

_____

_____

_____

_____

_____

_____

_____

Chapter Twelve

MAKING IT THROUGH THE BAD DAYS

If God hadn't been there for me, I never would have made it.
The minute I said, "I'm slipping, I'm falling,"
your love, God, took hold and held me fast.
When I was upset and beside myself,
you calmed me down and cheered me up.
—Psalm 94:17–19 *The Message*

More Waiting

During the second year of our wait, we learned that nearly all the families waiting to adopt had been chosen by birthparents—except us. —Sharon

"Adam, my arms ache to hold a child," said my bride Amy plaintively. "I know Peeps," I replied with sympathy. "But we have to wait on the Lord's timing." —Adam McManus

Be still before the Lord and wait patiently for him.
—Psalm 37:7

Kim's Journal

Dear God,
After the week of shots, we were ready for the three inseminations every other day during the time I should be ovulating, and then we waited. It seemed like an eternity before we could go back in for the pregnancy test.

Finally, the big day came to find out if I was going to be a mommy. The doctor came into the exam room and sadly informed us I wasn't pregnant. God, I couldn't believe what I was hearing! How could this be? We did everything we were supposed to! I was crushed. What will we do now? Not only can we not afford to do IUI again, I don't think our marriage would do too well. Was it all a waste?

I'm still going to the acupuncturist, obediently following the dietary plan, and taking prescribed vitamins. The months go by . . . and even after everything done to my body, I still can't ovulate or have a period. We're back at square one.
Crushed, Kim

A Mommy-in-Waiting Shares

After seven years of trying to get pregnant, our infertility diagnosis showed my husband was sterile. We pursued the traditional domestic adoption plan until God provided our adopted daughter.

Later, I heard a Focus on the Family radio program about the Snowflakes Embryo Adoption & Donation Program, which enables couples to carry a baby, my heart's lifelong desire. I called and requested the paperwork, and they matched us with a wonderful Christian couple who wanted to give their embryos a chance at life. Then the waiting *really* began. Almost daily for the next ten months, I called to check on the holdup. The donor couple was in the military, and there was a delay in releasing lab test results. —Mandy

Janet's Mentoring Moment

To quote Shannon, "The waiting is continuous!" Regardless of the route you choose to parenthood, you'll encounter a waiting period. God knew what you might resort to while waiting, so he advises in Matthew 6:27: "Who of you by worrying can add a single hour to his life?" Or create a life?

Shannon suggests doing nice things for yourself while you wait or when you receive disappointing news: go to tea, enjoy a massage, or take a trip together. Each spouse may have a different way of coping. Shannon always wants to take a getaway trip, and Dan would rather be around family.

Shannon also advises determining in advance who is going to receive "the news" if it comes via phone. Shannon opted for Dan to receive the calls and then present the results to her. Have this book open to Phone Notes, page 260, so you can write down everything that's said. You may be too emotional to remember, and you'll want all the details later.

God's Love Letter to You

*Dear*_____ *and*_____,

I, the LORD, long to be gracious to you; I rise to show you compassion. For I, the LORD, am a God of justice. Blessed are all who wait for me (Isa. 30:18, paraphrased)!
Waiting with you, God

Couple's Prayer

We waited patiently for you, LORD; you turned to us and heard our cry. You lifted us out of the slimy pit, out of the mud and mire; you set our feet on a rock and gave us a firm place to stand. You put a new song in our mouth, a hymn of praise to our God. Many will see and fear and put their trust in You, LORD. Amen. (Ps. 40:1–3, paraphrased)

THE JOURNEY CAN BE LONELY

Nothing compares to the extreme loneliness and worthlessness a barren woman feels. —Danette

The infertility experience has been an absolutely overwhelming and lonely experience. You cry until you think you can't cry any more, and then you cry some more. —Ann

TURN TO ME AND HAVE MERCY ON ME, BECAUSE I AM LONELY AND HURTING.
—Psalm 25:16 NCV

Kim's Journal

Dear God,
Shannon and I were experiencing infertility while our siblings, Sean and Michelle, already had children. It felt comforting knowing Toby and I weren't alone in our struggle. Shannon and Dan decided on IVF at the same time we decided on IUI, so going through that together was exciting. But when we received our results first that we weren't pregnant, I'm ashamed to admit I secretly wished the same fate for Shannon so I wouldn't be left behind, alone in my infertility.

When my mom called to tell me the news that Shannon and Dan were pregnant, I burst into tears. I didn't care who saw. My two officemates quietly left the room and closed the door. They didn't know what I'd just heard, but it must be horrible. My mom had breast cancer the year before, and I'm sure they thought she was dying.

I should've been happy for Shannon and Dan; they deserved to be parents as much as I thought we did. I just couldn't stop crying. I left work because I couldn't pull myself together. I knew only my mom would understand my reaction, so I went to her house. I had never felt so alone and needed to cry with someone.

Oh God, Shannon and Dan have successfully crossed over to the other side, leaving us behind in the dark. They're going to be parents . . . and we aren't. Life doesn't seem fair. We're the odd couple out in the family, and in that lonely place, I've succumbed to irrational jealousy.
Lonely, Kim

A Mommy-in-Waiting Shares

"Give me children, or I'll die," biblical Rachel cried to her husband Jacob as she watched her sister Leah give birth to baby after baby. "Remember me, Lord!" was the cry of Hannah's anguished heart as she wept before God. I can relate to feeling abandoned by God and wanting to die. If I as a woman couldn't pass any of me on through having a child, I might as well die now. It's the end of me anyway. Everywhere I go, women are pregnant or are already mothers. They talk about things I cannot understand and not because I don't want to. They have crossed over to this blessed land of fertility, and I've been left behind to dry up, alone!
—Danette

Janet's Mentoring Moment

In loneliness and despair, Kim hit rock bottom. If you've been there, you resonate with the feelings of abandonment when others cross over the goal line on the infertility journey. Jealousy often replaces camaraderie when a sojourner reaches her destination before you.

I was proud of Kim for not minimizing or rationalizing her jealousy. She knew the green envy monster had reared its ugly head, and only God could help her counter those harmful feelings. She confessed to God the sin of jealousy. She also didn't do the one thing she probably wanted to do—isolate. She still attended family functions and even went to Shannon's baby shower as God began softening her heart and helping her work through her feelings.

Hormones play a big role in irrational thinking, but succumbing to jealousy brings bitterness, not a baby. Even though you also may feel abandoned by God at the moment, he hasn't gone anywhere, and he's the only one who can comfort you. Sue Hawkes shares how she learned this truth in her article, "The Baby Club:"

After years of trying to have a baby, my husband and I realized it might never happen for us. As more and more babies piled into our church nursery, loneliness defined me. I wrestled with why God had chosen this path for us, and what, if not mothering, was my purpose in life. Eventually I realized what God was asking of me. I'd spent so much time and energy trying to fit in with the young moms at church, I'd neglected to hear God calling me closer to him. This was a turning point in my life. By allowing God to use this time in my life, I've discovered a depth of faith I'd never experienced before. God was teaching me that although I may feel alone, I don't need to feel lonely, because he's always with me.[1]

God's Love Letter to You

Dear_____ and_____,
You can be sure of this: I am with you always, even to the end of the age (Matt. 28:20b NLT, paraphrased).
Your constant companion, God

Couple's Prayer

God, Where are you? When is it going to be our turn? We need to feel your presence. We feel empty and alone, and we don't like the thoughts we're having about others whom you've blessed with children. If you're not going to give us children right now, what do you want us to do? Give us pure minds and hearts. Protect us from the evils of jealousy and coveting. We're begging you. Amen.

IT'S HARD BEING BRAVE

The most difficult part for me was constantly having to be happy for other people. —Karen

I TRY TO MAKE THE BEST OF IT, TRY TO BRAVE IT OUT.
—Job 10:16 *The Message*

Shannon's Journal

Dear God,
A week after our positive pregnancy test, I was lying in bed when suddenly the pain became unbearable. I thought I had appendicitis. We rushed to the emergency room where an

ultrasound showed I was having an ectopic pregnancy—one of the embryos had gone into my fallopian tube, and they had to operate. Oh Lord, I was so afraid. What if I lost all the embryos, and what would the surgery do to the others? I couldn't believe this was happening . . . it seemed like everything was going so well, and now this. I couldn't stop crying, but I wanted to be brave for my other babies.

When I woke up from surgery and learned they removed my right fallopian tube with the embryo, I felt like our chances of getting pregnant in the future had been cut in half. The doctor said a second embryo had "sloughed off," but the remaining embryo had attached and was looking good.

Oh God, trying to get pregnant has been traumatic enough without this happening. But I'm praising you for the baby we still have. Please don't let the surgery cause him or her any problems. Help this baby hang on . . . make him, or her, a fighter!

Bravely, Shannon

A Mommy-in-Waiting Shares

Shannon's "little fighter," our grandson Joshua, did hold on and was born on Father's Day. The following Christmas, Kim tried being brave during what she described as "the worst Christmas of my life."

I knew it was going to be especially hard this Christmas. Shannon had her baby now, and I was still in waiting. I had never felt jealous or envious of my siblings and their families during the holidays in the past. I really enjoyed being an aunt and spending time with my nieces and nephews. But this Christmas was different; now we were the *only* couple without a "family." I felt small and lonely as Toby and I sat watching the craziness of children opening gifts all around us. We opened our gifts, watching as the gift giving among the children continued for what seemed an eternity. It was like being an outsider watching somebody else's family. I felt alone in a house full of people, noise, and excitement. —Kim

Janet's Mentoring Moment

Every infertility story is fraught with times of great sorrow, emotional pain, and breakdowns. You're going to have bad days. Often Christians think they must remain strong and brave at *all* times, and any indication of sadness shows a lack of faith. Not true. In the Bible, the psalmists' faith allows them to cry out to God for comfort when they're not feeling strong and brave. You'll read and pray many psalms in this book.

It's not healthy living in a constant state of denial with repressed feelings. God provided the gift of tears because he knew we would need to express our pain. Tears are cleansing and healing. They're God's plan for pent-up emotions to escape before spewing. The world looks cleaner and brighter after a good, soul-cleansing cry.

You may need to put on a happy face at work or for other children. Your family and friends, especially children, may be frightened when you cry or have outbursts. Find a secluded refuge, even if it's locked in the bathroom, and cry, rant at God, and ask "Why?" Inform loved ones that when you cry or don't feel like being cheery, it's the time you need their compassion and love the most.

God's Love Letter to You

Dear_____ and_____,
Be brave. Be strong. Don't give up. Expect me, God, to arrive soon (Ps. 31:24 *The Message,* paraphrased).
Catching each tear, God

Couple's Prayer

Lord, We long to be like Job who told his wife, "We take the good days from God—why not also the bad days?" (Job 2:10 *The Message*). We want to be godly representatives, but we're hurting. This ordeal is so difficult, and our hearts break thinking of all we must endure. We just want to have kids like everyone else. Help us be strong when we need to be. Thank you for understanding and giving us the blessing of tears. Amen.

SURVIVING THE HOLIDAYS

Holidays were heart-wrenching. Mother's Day and Father's Day were the worst. —Sharon

I remember sending my mom a Mother's Day card and lamenting that nobody would ever do that for me. I love my mother so much and she is a dear friend. So the idea of no one ever having those thoughts about me, loving me that way, calling me Mommy, killed me inside. —Danette

WHY DOES YOUR FACE LOOK SO SAD WHEN YOU ARE NOT ILL?
THIS CAN BE NOTHING BUT SADNESS OF HEART.
—Nehemiah 2:2

Kim's Journal

Dear God,

It's almost Mother's Day, and I don't know if I can handle seeing all those happy moms at church and brunch. I'm trying to focus on my mom and not think about how I'm missing out on being a mommy on yet another Mother's Day. This year is especially hard since we've been trying to be parents for so long and so hard, only to be repeatedly disappointed.

At the store looking for a card for my mom, I see the cute "To Mommy" cards at the end of the aisle . . . oh God, I wish I were someone's mommy! I look away and continue focusing on the task ahead, getting my mom and mothers-in-law their cards.

Today's the day: it's Mother's Day. I don't think I can bear it. It's just begun and already I want this day over. I pull myself out of bed and get ready for church. I'm not looking forward to the sermon about children being a blessing and honoring mothers. God, help me focus on *my* mom.

We met my parents at church and I put on my happy face, when inside I was crying watching all the mothers with big smiles dressed in pretty spring dresses and children running all around. This was a day of celebration, and I just wanted to go back to bed. The pastor started the message with asking all the mothers to stand up. Hundreds of women stood and everyone applauded. I couldn't take it any longer and sat slouched over in my seat, quietly crying. Toby put his arm around me and my mom held my hand, but nothing took away the pain. I barely heard the rest of the message.

After brunch, I came home, collapsed on my bed, and cried myself to sleep, where I remained the rest of the day. God, please don't make me go through another Mother's Day with this hole in my heart. I want to stand up in church with all those other mothers beaming from ear to ear and have everyone applaud me. God, please let me stand up next year.

Desperate to be a mommy, Kim

A Mommy-in-Waiting Shares

On Mother's Day our pastor said, "Sons are a heritage from the Lord, children a reward from him." Why wasn't I rewarded and blessed? I was focusing my anger and frustration on God. I hear other women complain about being pregnant . . . again! In the news, there are stories about unwed mothers abandoning their babies or the rising numbers of abortions. All this tragedy, why couldn't God bless me with a baby? To make matters worse, all of my sisters-in-law and my own sister were pregnant! —Gay Lynne

Janet's Mentoring Moment

On Mother's Day and Father's Day, it's difficult for friends, family, and churches to know how to honor parents without hurting those who aren't parents. One year our church downplayed Mother's Day and didn't have mothers stand up. As a mother, I felt overlooked. I'm sure other mothers felt the same way, especially those who, like Kim, had been waiting for the day when they could jump out of their seats.

The next year, the church resumed the tradition of having mothers stand, but first acknowledged that there were many in the congregation who had lost a mother or were longing for a child, and they prayed for them before celebrating the moms. Today, the church takes pictures of *all* the women on Mother's Day—a nice, inclusive way for every woman to feel acknowledged.

All family-gathering holidays and reunions are difficult. Don't feel you have to forge ahead with a smile on your face and not admit that it's a tough day for you. Find tips for surviving the holidays on page 269.

God's Love Letter to You

Dear_____ and_____,
Go home and prepare a feast, holiday food and drink; and share it with those who don't have anything: This day is holy to God. Don't feel bad. The joy of God is your strength (Neh. 8:10 *The Message*)!
Your strength, God

Couple's Prayer

Father, We call you Father when we ourselves so long to be parents. The holidays rub salt into our wounds and empty womb. Help us take the focus off our own pain as we celebrate with others a day that is special to so many. We want to find hope in knowing this day will pass, and perhaps you have a holiday full of joy planned for us in the future. Let us celebrate our own love for each other on holidays, and most importantly, celebrate how much you love us. Amen.

HUSBANDS HAVE BAD DAYS, TOO

At times it seemed the pain of watching Jeff hurting was greater than my own pain. I heard one woman say her husband had never felt more like a man than when he had gotten her pregnant. I hated the thought that I couldn't fix this for Jeff and he couldn't fix it for me. —Danette

AS IRON SHARPENS IRON, SO ONE MAN SHARPENS ANOTHER.
—Proverbs 27:17

Kim's Journal

Dear God,

I know that even though Toby shows his emotions differently than I do, he's struggling with not having a baby and my constant emotional breakdowns. He hates to see me hurting and not be able to help. He's uncomfortable with the infertility treatment program and says getting tested is so embarrassing. I think he's ready to drop the whole idea.

It helped when he and Dan could talk about things together, but when Shannon got pregnant, those conversations stopped. God, please bring another couple into our lives we can talk to or a husband who understands what Toby's going through. I know he prays and talks to you. Please comfort him, especially when I'm too caught up in my own emotions to be there for him.

A concerned wife, Kim

A Daddy-in-Waiting Shares

Sharing our grief, disappointment, and disillusionment with other couples experiencing the same things helped us during our infertility. Through mutual sharing, my wife was able to verbalize with others that it wasn't pregnancy she craved, but motherhood. Also around this time, several years into the infertility process, I began to relate more fully to the incredible passion my wife had for a family. To a greater extent than before, her passion began to become my passion. —Dan, Gay Lynne's husband

Janet's Mentoring Moment

A Daddy-in-Waiting feels alone and isolated from other men in his family and circle of friends. It's difficult talking about infertility and insecurity issues unless it's with another man experiencing something similar. Dan and Toby spoke freely to each other about the testing and procedures, but it wasn't a topic of conversation among their buddies or at work.

Men need to confide in other men just like women need to confide in other women. Make a conscious effort to form relationships with other couples in support groups, at doctors' offices, or at adoption agencies and invite them over for dinner or out to coffee for a chat. You know what always happens: the women start talking to each other, and then the men start talking, and soon their discussion moves from sports to common issues.

Don't overlook a husband's feelings, insecurities, fears, opinions, wishes, and desires. He may have trouble verbalizing his uneasiness or concerns, but he's part of the team. Occasionally he's going to need a shoulder to cry on, too—be sure it's a healthy, appropriate shoulder. He may want to consider participating in a men's group at church.

God's Love Letter to You

Dear_____ and_____,
Go home to your own [family and relatives and friends] and bring back word to them of how much I, the Lord, have done for you, and [how I] had sympathy for you and mercy on you (Mark 5:19 AMP, paraphrased).
Man-to-Man, God

Couple's Prayer

Father, We pray for you to bring into our life another couple dealing with infertility, who has your perspective on our plight. If you're asking us to step out and be that comfort to someone else, make us willing and ready. Especially for me, the husband, I need this, Lord. I'm admitting I can't get through this on my own. I need your help. Please bring me Jesus in skin. Amen.

Your Letter to God

There's no denying that an infertility journey includes numerous "bad" days. With God's love and strength, you'll make it through. Talk to God about tough days, and ask him to show you ways to minimize their negative impact. It's OK to cry out and to cry.

Dear God,_____ Date:_____

_____

_____

_____

_____

_____

_____

_____

_____

_____

_____

_____

_____

_____

_____

_____

_____

_____

_____

Chapter Thirteen

KNOWING WHO IS IN CONTROL

My very dear friends, when you see people
reducing God to something they can use or control,
get out of their company as fast as you can.
—1 Corinthians 10:14 *The Message*

Spinning Out of Control

After our twin girls died, I couldn't look at pregnant women. If anyone I knew had a baby, I started crying. I couldn't attend baby showers. I got pregnant again, but I lost it at about four weeks. I was on an emotional rollercoaster. —Marissa

Those who do not control themselves are like a city whose walls are broken down.
—Proverbs 25:28 NCV

Kim's Journal

Dear God,

Shannon's pregnancy was harder on me than anyone else's. When my cousin found out she was pregnant, I felt a pang of resentment toward her happiness, but it wasn't overwhelming jealousy. Since Shannon and I had experienced infertility together, I felt abandoned. She had victoriously achieved her goal, and I hadn't. I lost it. I was at my lowest point, completely irrational. How could I pretend to be happy for her, when all I wanted to do was cry? I was so angry with you, God . . . didn't you see what great parents Toby and I would be?

When I finally did see Shannon, her belly already was showing. Thanks, God! How was I supposed to avoid the subject when it was staring me in the face? It turns out the hormones caused bloating, making her appear further along than she was. I put on my happy face and congratulated her.

The next few days for Shannon were pretty rough. She lost one of the babies, and a second traveled up into a fallopian tube, requiring surgical removal and leaving her with only one fallopian tube and one baby. My heart began to soften and change. This must have been such a difficult time for her, and all I could think about was *myself*. I prayed for Shannon's health and the baby she was left carrying.

I know, God, that you have a plan. I don't know what it is for me, but I can't hold this little miracle baby you've blessed Shannon with accountable for my own hurts. Please help me get my emotions under control. Wash away my irrational jealousy, and open up my heart to love this innocent child you created.

Out of control, Kim

A Mommy-in-Waiting Shares

The most emotionally devastating moment came when I had to have an ultrasound for a medical study after the implantation failed. There on the monitor was the image of my empty womb. My husband Daniel understood that most of the procedures happened to my body, but he said, "I don't want us not to try again because of fear." He promised to abide by my decision.

While I was deciding, a guest speaker at church spoke about infertility issues with his wife. Our pastor had an altar call for those who were angry with God to repent and receive forgiveness. I'd been sitting in the pew the last few weeks thinking I had to find a way to hold on to God, or everything I had was going to fall apart. I couldn't get to the altar fast enough.

Out of love for Daniel, I tried again. The doctor gave me a different regimen of fertility medications, and I responded quickly and phenomenally. They harvested about twenty-six eggs and were able to implant the two best fertilized embryos. —Melanie

Janet's Mentoring Moment

Every infertility story has some element of spinning out of control. Emotions are raw, and the wife's hormones run rapid. The husband is also dealing with potential loss of fatherhood and pressure from not continuing the family line. Both experience an emotional rollercoaster of highs . . . lows . . . hopefulness . . . disappointment . . . anticipation . . . anxiety . . . fear.

Fear births angry doubts while eroding confidence in God. You've probably said or felt: I'm *afraid* I'll never have a baby. I'm *afraid* having a baby isn't God's plan for us. I'm *afraid* the procedure won't work. I'm *afraid* the birthmother will change her mind. Even if you didn't verbalize the word *afraid,* fear was behind every "Why?" and desperate emotion and action.

Fear ignites out-of-control feelings, resulting in the compelling need to take control. We say to God, "Fix it, or else!" Max Lucado confirms, "Fear, at its center, is a perceived loss of control. When life spins wildly, we grab for a component of life we can manage: our diet, the tidiness of a house, the armrest of a plane, or, in many cases, people. The more insecure we feel, the meaner we become. We growl and bare our fangs."[1] Does that describe you lately?

On your own, you can't control fear, but God can. Even if you're angry with God, be real with him because he already knows how you're feeling—he's God. Ask for his help. You can't stay on a rollercoaster for long without losing your balance, equilibrium, and maybe your lunch; you can't stay in an emotional, out-of-control state for long, either. Soon everything and everyone will upset you, and the onslaught of emotions could destroy all that you hold dear.

Going through a crisis without God is like being on a rollercoaster that never stops until it crashes. If you don't have God at the center of your life, go to page 245 and pray the prayer that will stop your world from spinning out of control. If God is in your life, give him back the controls. Do you feel your feet getting back on the ground? Steady now, you might still be a bit shaky.

God's Love Letter to You

Dear_____ and_____,

Do not be afraid, for I am with you and will bless you (Gen. 26:24 NLT).

In control of the universe, God

Couple's Prayer

Lord, We detest feeling as if we're losing our sanity. We ask the Holy Spirit living within us to help us regain stability in our emotions and actions. As dark as things seem, we want to believe it won't be like this forever. We trust your plan for our lives, and we know the stress and upheaval we're experiencing isn't getting us any further toward our goal of parenthood. We're breathing in the Holy Spirit and exhaling out the friction and pain that has been consuming us. Thank you for the peace that only you can provide. Amen.

CONTROLLING THE CONTROLLABLE

I remember it well. Like any woman who is "in control" and awaiting a planned pregnancy, I lived my life in two-week increments—waiting to ovulate or waiting to see if I was pregnant. It really is quite maddening, but exciting at the same time. —Karen

IF I KEEP MY EYES ON GOD, I WON'T TRIP OVER MY OWN FEET.
—Psalm 25:15 *The Message*

Kim's Journal

Dear God,

Well, we've been trying for a year to have a baby, and now Toby's career is relocating us four hours away from home. I'm quitting work to be a stay-at-home wife and . . . hopefully some-day . . . a mother. That was our original plan, and we're sticking with it. We haven't decided what we're going to do next after our failed attempt at IUI. Toby's insurance won't cover as much as mine did. I'll have to find a new fertility doctor and start over again if we choose that path.

When we first set out on this fertility assistance process, we prayed about the direction you wanted us going. I'm not sure we ever heard you telling us to do the artificial insemina-tion, but we so desperately wanted to be parents, and why wouldn't you want that for us, too? We felt IUI wasn't far from your natural process—we were just "helping" the process along through technology. But you spoke clearly that we weren't to explore any of the more advanced fertility treatments. So we've decided to stop trying to control conception and open our minds to other options, such as adoption.

We want parenthood more than pregnancy. If it isn't meant for me to give birth to a child, then you must have a bigger plan for our lives.

Surrendering control, Kim

Two Mommies-in-Waiting Share

During the first IVF, we inserted all five embryos and *none* of them attached! That was a rude, sad awakening. It was the first thing in my life I couldn't control. I could make things happen at work, but I couldn't make myself get pregnant. I had assumed IVF would work like the doctor said and fix our infertility problem.

When it didn't, I began wondering if it wasn't God's will or plan for us to have a baby.

I hadn't prayed much about getting pregnant, but now I prayed to God for answers. My previous prayers had been for God to bless my work or help me make a sale. Now I asked, "Is having a baby your will for my life?" I was young in my faith when we started this process, but our failed first attempt at IVF grew me closer to the Lord. —Paula

꙰

I'm a control freak. I thought I'd come off the pill and get pregnant. After all, I'm in control of my body. Infertility was a spiritual learning process of God teaching me I wasn't in control of my body—God was. I don't regret the journey because it put me flat on my face praying and pleading to God daily for a year and a half. —Melissa

Janet's Mentoring Moment

Kay Warren has a mantra I quoted in my book *Dear God, They Say It's Cancer*: "I want to control the controllable and leave the uncontrollable to God." As much as we might try to embrace this practice, we often take back things as fast as we give them to God.

As you continue reading, you'll see how in control God was in Kim's and Shannon's lives and in those of the couples sharing their stories. God had the solutions for parenthood; their job was to trust and obey him. Even when you face the unexpected in life, it's never unexpected to God. Ask God to reveal your part in his sovereign plan, and he'll do the rest.

God's Love Letter to You

Dear_____ and_____,
My grace is sufficient for you, for my power is made perfect in weakness (2 Cor. 12:9a).
Your stronghold, God

Couple's Prayer

Lord, You are omnipotent. Therefore we will boast all the more gladly about our weaknesses, so that Christ's power may rest on us. That is why, for Christ's sake, we delight in weaknesses, in insults, in hardships, in persecutions, in difficulties. For when we are weak, then we are strong. Amen. (2 Cor. 12:9b–10, paraphrased)

TEMPTATIONS AND DISTRACTIONS

In my anxiety, pushing every direction to get a child, trying to be in good shape, and being in control (NOT!), I was thrust into a waterskiing accident which almost resulted in the removal of my left lower leg. —Mandy

KEEP WATCH AND PRAY, SO THAT YOU WILL NOT GIVE IN TO TEMPTATION. FOR THE SPIRIT IS WILLING, BUT THE BODY IS WEAK!
—Matthew 26:41 NLT

Kim's Journal

Dear God,

We were making a big move and ready for a fresh start. Before we ventured too far into the adoption thought, we received a call from the fertility clinic. They were conducting a study on eggs, and if we participated, we would receive a free IVF cycle. Wow! Couples would kill for this opportunity. IVF was expensive, and to have it *totally* covered was unimaginable.

Just when we were starting to hear your voice in this whole process, here came a huge temptation to take back control of our situation. We prayed hard. Was this from you or was it a distraction? Our new home was four hours away from the fertility clinic. We knew what we had to do. You had made it clear from the beginning that IVF wasn't your plan for us.

So we turned down the offer, but they had *another* offer. Someone had donated "meds," and we could do another insemination cycle with free meds. Still not sure if your hand was in this, we decided to go forward with one more try at IUI. I justified the long drive to the clinic as an excuse to go back home and visit my mom.

Second-guessing, Kim

A Mommy-in-Waiting Shares

Simon and I are one flesh in God's eyes, and we agreed donor insemination would be circumventing God's plans for us. Just because I can have children naturally, while Simon can't, doesn't mean I should do so, but it's not easy dismissing that option. I still think about DI occasionally; however, feelings of discomfort or disagreement never go away. I think if God were telling me to pursue that option, I wouldn't have those niggling doubts. I realize that wanting to pursue DI stems from my own selfish hopes, reasons, and desires, which I'm still trying to align with God's desires and hopes for us.

After much prayer and information gathering, we decided on frozen embryo adoption. The hundreds of thousands of lives frozen in storage labs waiting to be born tugged at our hearts. Regardless of how these lives were created, shouldn't they have a chance at life before we, who aren't able to produce our own children, try to create more on our own? Only *one* embryo survived the thawing process for implantation, but to our delight, we were officially pregnant with a Caucasian baby, not Chinese like us. —Tiffany

Janet's Mentoring Moment

On your journey, you'll encounter subtle and enticing temptations to detour off the Family Plan and the parameters you developed together on page 256. Your plan should be flexible, but many couples encounter a crossroads where they're trying to discern if it's their own will or God's will they're pursuing. Maybe it's a free treatment opportunity—how can you turn that down, you think—yet you wonder what God thinks.

Maybe your plan was to leave no stone unturned and keep trying procedures until you run out of money or time. If you're in agreement with that path and believe it's God's plan, then keep going. But if either of you feels enough is enough, it's time to reconsider. Peace in *both* your hearts is the key to knowing God's will. If either of you has nagging doubts, God is trying to get your attention.

God's Love Letter to You

Dear_____ and_____,
No test or temptation that comes your way is beyond the course of what others have had to face. All you need to remember is that I, God, will never let you down; I'll never let you be pushed past your limit; I'll always be there to help you come through it (1 Cor. 10:13 *The Message*, paraphrased).
Your Overcomer, God

Couple's Prayer

Lord, We're asking you to direct our path and keep it straight on the road that leads to the fulfillment of your plans. You know how badly we want to be parents, and we admit we're tempted to try anything and everything that comes our way. Provide us with discernment to identify what is from you and what is a distraction. Options, or lack of them, torment us. We find comfort in knowing none of this is a surprise to you. Calm our hearts. Remove our anxiety.

Give us clear vision. Invade our souls with peace and let us stay confidently united in our thoughts and prayers. Amen.

TAKING BACK CONTROL

I remember questioning everything in my life: my marriage, schooling, career choice. I was searching for something to grab onto that would explain why pregnancy wasn't happening for us. I would obsess about the things I could control because there was so much I couldn't control.

—Shannon

TEACH ME TO DO WHAT YOU WANT, BECAUSE YOU ARE MY GOD.
LET YOUR GOOD SPIRIT LEAD ME ON LEVEL GROUND.
—Psalm 143:10 NCV

Kim's Journal

Dear God,

Shortly after settling into our new home, we started round two of IUI, and I began the long drives back to Orange County to the fertility clinic every other day. Sometimes I stayed overnight with Mom, but usually I'd start out early, go to my appointment, and head back home. Toby worked out of his company's Southern California office when he needed to deliver his specimen. I was exhausted from driving, but we were making it work. Then Toby started feeling unsure about the shots. He didn't think he could do them again.

I was so excited we'd been given one more opportunity that I couldn't let anything stand in my way. I'd learn how to give myself the shots. This was a huge deal, since I've been known to pass out at the sight of blood. Thankfully, the needle was smaller than before. I felt confident I could do it. The first night, Toby loaded the syringe and got everything ready. Wow, I was really going to stick a needle into myself. God, I prayed you would give me the strength and courage. Toby sat next to me and rubbed my neck.

OK, here I go. One, two, three, stick! I pressed down on the syringe, depositing the contents into my stomach, removed the needle, and pressed the area with an alcohol pad Toby had ready. It wasn't as bad as I expected. I could do this. Since I could see what I was doing, I didn't feel the nervous anticipation of waiting for that big needle to come from behind. By the third night, I quietly administered the shot in the bathroom and slipped into bed. Toby asked if we were ready to do the shots, and I told him it was done.

Without the stress of the shots, we were more at ease this time around, even with the added driving. More relaxed, I was sure of success at creating a baby. God, thank you for the courage to give myself shots. You know our hearts and our desires. Please fulfill our dream to be parents.

Under control, Kim

A Mommy-in-Waiting Shares

During a special weekend at church, we were challenged to allow God to have full control of our lives—wants, hopes, and desires—by writing on a piece of paper whatever we were holding back from God, tear it up, and leave it on the worship center altar. I knew God wanted me to put the pregnancy issue on the altar, and when I did, it was more than symbolic. I truly was able to give God my heart in this issue.

I realized for the first time it wasn't up to me whether I ever had a baby. I also was able to say it was all right either way, and I meant it. I did ask God to take away my desire for children if that wasn't His plan for us. As long as I had the desire, I believed one day He would answer our prayers. But God's plan for our marriage and our lives was the most important thing, not whether or not we became parents. The bitterness drained out of my heart and left assurance that God was in control. Leaving my burden on that altar began a journey of spiritual transformation that continues to this day.[2] —Chris Adams, "My Struggle with Infertility"

Janet's Mentoring Moment

Kim gave up control and then took it back, but Chris Adams experienced the freedom that comes from complete surrender. No matter how much we *think* we're in control of our life, destiny, circumstances, resources, options, plans—our world—we're not! God is. God controls everything in the universe, and often he needs to remind us of his omniscience. When we're trying to control a situation, we're literally trying to do God's job, and he'll never let us replace him, though many try.

In a crisis, we're willing to sacrifice everything for his intervention. We cry out, begging him to take control over the situation, but what he wants most is for us to grant him authority over our self-will. We want him to fix what we can't fix, but he wants to fix us. Relinquishing complete control to God requires allowing his will to be done in our life as it is in heaven.

God's Love Letter to You

Dear_____ and_____,

Who took charge of the ocean when it gushed forth like a baby from the womb? That was me! I wrapped it in soft clouds, and tucked it in safely at night. Then I made a playpen for it, a strong playpen so it couldn't run loose, and said, "Stay here, this is your place. Your wild tantrums are confined to this place." And have you ever ordered Morning, "Get up!" or told Dawn, "Get to work!" (Job 38:8–12 *The Message*)?

In charge, God

Couple's Prayer

Lord, It's hard not making this all about us, when it really should be all about you! We do try to take back the reins from you. Help us remember we don't have to be in control. You have everything under your great and mighty, controlling, righteous right hand, in which we can rest assured that even though we can't see what you're doing, it'll all turn out well. Amen.

SURRENDERING CONTROL

When I look back and see everything I went through, I can see that it was under God's control all along. —Gay Lynne

No longer could I try to "plan" my life or my family. It was too much for me to handle. I was too broken and didn't even want to try to be in control any longer. I gave it all over to God. —Michele

LET THE MORNING BRING ME WORD OF YOUR UNFAILING LOVE,
FOR I HAVE PUT MY TRUST IN YOU. SHOW ME THE WAY I SHOULD GO,
FOR TO YOU I LIFT UP MY SOUL.
—Psalm 143:8

Shannon's Journal

Dear God,

When I can't sleep or I cry so much it hurts, I turn on praise music or get out my journal and ask you "Why?" Sometimes, I just lie on the floor looking up, cry, tell you how bad it hurts, and ask you to show me what to do. I ask you to heal me. I surrender all my pain to you.

You often send a song, a person, or a word in my devotion or prayer time, and I know you're with me lifting the burden and pain I feel in the moment. I write down in my journal what you send me as your promises, and I hold on to them. I ask you a question, and I'm amazed

how quickly you send an answer or something to comfort me and give me peace. It may not always be right away, but I remind myself that tomorrow when I wake up, I may feel better.
Giving up control, Shannon

Two Mommies-in-Waiting Share

Originally, my husband Ron's opinion of adoption was "absolutely not" and "I don't want someone else's child." But as Ron prayerfully became more open to the idea, I got a bit excited about this new "treatment" and started pursuing adoption agencies. Slowly, we began realizing we had no control over the fact of being infertile or our intent to adopt, so we gave it all to the Lord.

Instead of asking him for a child, we asked that his will be done his way and that he use our experiences to bring about something good. We started believing he really does know what's best. Then, after nine years of infertility and approaching our fortieth birthdays, we received "the call" from the adoption agency. A birthmother requested a childless couple—we were the longest waiting childless couple. We knew God was in complete control. As we prepared to leave the hospital with our two-day-old baby girl, we realized if we had given up at *any* point on the journey, we wouldn't have her. We were utterly amazed at how the Lord places the right child into the right family and works out all the details and circumstances. —Sharon

During my deepest pain, our preacher shared a sermon titled "The Bitter and the Sweet." If God wants something for you, he'll work it out and it will be "sweet." When we do things our way without trusting that God knows best, we're in for a "bitter" situation. With blind trust, I peaceably and totally surrendered *my* will to *his* during that sermon. The pain completely left my heart. The want was still there, but the ache of the missing child was gone. It was OK with me if God's plan was for me to be barren. Little did I know that while my heart was undergoing this transformation, a little blond-haired, blue-eyed baby boy was being born about sixty miles west. —Robin

Janet's Mentoring Moment

All the couples in this book saw God at work when they let him do his work. Every story tells of surrendering control to God. You'll read later the incredible blessing God had for Kim and Toby when they finally surrendered control completely, and his will became their will.

Shannon said that in her darkest hours she called out to God, and he always presented himself to her through other people, a song, a prayer, or reading his Word. Are you looking for God when you call to him? He's there, and if you seek him, you'll find him.

Shannon also mentioned seeing God at work through journaling. Those who shared their stories for this book will never forget the glorious work of the Lord because they have it in writing. If you haven't been journaling in the space provided, go back now and write your Love Letters to God. Also use the Prayer & Praise Journal, page 272. Your faith will be strengthened as you see the mighty hand of the Lord in your life. Circumstances aren't random happenings. When there seems to be no way, God *always* makes a way—his way.

God's Love Letter to You

Dear_____and_____,

Trust me, God, from the bottom of your heart; don't try to figure out everything on your own (Prov. 3:5 *The Message,* paraphrased).

Always in control, God

Couple's Prayer

Abba, Father, we're giving all our hopes and dreams of having a child to you. We've been holding on tightly to our wants and ways, and we've only met dead ends and disappointments. You have our attention, Father. We surrender. We're broken in all the right places, and we're ready to do things your way. Amen.

Your Letter to God

Have you surrendered control of your life to God? If so, write about it so you can return and read what you wrote when you're tempted to take back the reins. If you haven't completely surrendered control, then tell God what's stopping you. List out-of-control areas, and cross off everything you can't do anything to change. Feel the reins slipping out of your hands.

Dear God,_____   Date:_____

_____

_____

_____

Chapter Fourteen

GRIEVING THE LOSSES

I AM BENT OVER AND RACKED WITH PAIN.
MY DAYS ARE FILLED WITH GRIEF.
I AM EXHAUSTED AND COMPLETELY CRUSHED.
MY GROANS COME FROM AN ANGUISHED HEART.
YOU KNOW WHAT I LONG FOR, LORD;
YOU HEAR MY EVERY SIGH.
—Psalm 38:6, 8–9 NLT

Crying Out to God

Grief deepens you: I'm a different person on the other side of it. I'm humbled and more sensitive, and I believe my trust in God has deepened. Once you experience grief, you aren't as rattled by it next time because you've experienced that when you cry out to God, he meets you where you're at, and you know he'll be there again no matter what happens. It's also a season in life that will pass, and a happier season is usually around the corner. —Shannon

I CALL TO GOD, I CRY TO GOD TO HELP ME. FROM HIS PALACE HE HEARS MY CALL; MY CRY BRINGS ME RIGHT INTO HIS PRESENCE—A PRIVATE AUDIENCE!
—Psalm 18:6 *The Message*

Kim's Journal

Dear God,
We were so optimistic during the second round of IUI. Toby's sperm count was great, and my body responded well to the hormones. If it was ever going to happen, this should have been the time. All conditions were perfect. So when we received the news from the doctor's office that we still weren't pregnant, we were devastated. How could this be? If we couldn't get pregnant under these circumstances, then we were never going to be parents.

I felt empty. I mourned the baby I'd never have growing inside me. Curled up in a ball on the floor and hugging my barren womb, I cried out to you, God: Why does it seem like people a

lot less "ready" than I am are able to have children . . . women out of wedlock . . . teenagers . . . drug addicts . . . felons? I'm a normal, happily married, middle class Christian woman who desperately wants to be a mother. There's something seriously wrong here! God, I don't know what your plan is, but surely it isn't for me never to be a mother.
Crying out, Kim

A Mommy-in-Waiting Shares

The way I grieve the loss of the babies is to be alone in my room, cry out to God, weep with my husband, journal all my feelings to Jesus, read the Scriptures he leads me to, and sleep. It takes a good three days. My husband is good about running the house while I'm grieving. He doesn't expect much from me, thankfully, and he may bring home my favorite food for dinner. I just need time to rest from emotional exhaustion. —Mandy

Janet's Mentoring Moment

When you're grieving, God is the person to cry out to. The night before his crucifixion, Jesus also cried out. "'I feel bad enough right now to die,'. . . He fell to the ground and prayed for a way out: 'Papa, Father, you can—can't you?—get me out of this. Take this cup away from me'" (Mark 14:34–36 *The Message*). Again at the cross, Jesus cried, "My God, my God, why have you forsaken me?" (Mark 15:34).

God hadn't forsaken Jesus and he hasn't forsaken you. He was in Jesus at the cross and he's in you in your infertility. Jesus prayed for a different way, but he also added, "Yet I want your will to be done, not mine" (Mark 14:36 NLT). Can you pray that, too? God didn't substitute an alternate plan to spare Jesus from going through pain. God heard Jesus, but he had no Plan B for saving the world. He knew Jesus' anguish, but he also knew the coming victory. This might not comfort you now, but God is involved in your pain even though he may seem painfully distant. He's still working on his Plan A for you.

God's Love Letter to You

Dear_____ and_____,
As each night watch begins, get up and cry out in prayer. Pour your heart out face-to-face with me, your Master (Lam. 2:19 *The Message*, paraphrased). If you do cry out to me, I will certainly hear your cry (Exod. 22:23, paraphrased).
I hear you, God

Couple's Prayer

Abba, Father, it's with clenched fists and teeth and through our tears that we say: let your will be done in our lives. We don't like the way things are going, and we can't imagine anything good coming out of this wretched pain, but we have the hope that your Plan A for us is a good one. Until we see that plan unfold, please help us hang on to you and to each other. Make your presence visible in our lives. We need you, Lord. We're crying out to you. Amen.

FEELING GUILTY

I struggled with thoughts that the miscarriages were my fault. Somehow I was to blame. Perhaps I was being punished by God for not being worthy enough to have a family or a good enough Christian. —Michele

Sometimes I feel an unwelcome sense of guilt because parenthood often is treated as a superior status in society. Or because we didn't get a second mortgage for IVF, some would say we didn't try hard enough! —Rachel L.

YOU'LL BE ABLE TO FACE THE WORLD UNASHAMED AND KEEP A FIRM GRIP ON LIFE, GUILTLESS AND FEARLESS. YOU'LL FORGET YOUR TROUBLES; THEY'LL BE LIKE OLD, FADED PHOTOGRAPHS. YOUR WORLD WILL BE WASHED IN SUNSHINE, EVERY SHADOW DISPERSED BY DAYSPRING. FULL OF HOPE, YOU'LL RELAX, CONFIDENT AGAIN; YOU'LL LOOK AROUND, SIT BACK, AND TAKE IT EASY.
—Job 11:15–19 *The Message*

Kim's Journal

Dear God,
Why are you doing this to me? Why don't you want me to have a baby? I feel guilty for my jealousy and feeling like an outsider in my own family. Is that the reason you're not giving us a baby?
Guiltily, Kim

A Mommy-in-Waiting Shares

After my miscarriage, I felt awkward seeing all the young families at church. One couple, Gina and John, were pregnant, and every time I saw Gina's growing tummy, I envied her. I knew she was at least eight years younger than me; it just wasn't fair. As soon as we got the green light to try again, we dragged the fertility monitor out of the closet. We were pleasantly surprised to be pregnant after only two months.

Then, horrible news: Gina and John lost their baby three weeks before his delivery date. I was overwhelmed with guilt. To think of how I had struggled with so much envy and jealousy toward Gina, and now I couldn't fathom her pain. I grieved for them. —Michele

Janet's Mentoring Moment

Guilt is a phase of grieving that can happen at any stage of the journey. Maybe you feel guilty for things in your past or envying others or feeling better when someone else struggles, too. Perhaps you finally get pregnant and feel guilty about the others who didn't. Or you wonder if you tried hard and long enough before changing to another option.

Guilt isn't from God. Remorse, repentance, forgiveness are God's terms. Satan uses guilt to destroy you and your relationships. If you need to confess jealousy, go directly to the person and ask for his or her forgiveness. If you feel you've sinned against God, ask him for forgiveness. Then enjoy the heart-filled love and compassion for others that God feels for you.

God's Love Letter to You

Dear_____ and_____,
Make a careful exploration of who you are and the work you have been given, and then sink yourself into that. Don't be impressed with yourself. Don't compare yourself with others. Each of you must take responsibility for doing the creative best you can with your own life (Gal. 6:4–5 The Message).
Freeing you of guilt, God

Couple's Prayer

Father, We know guilt isn't from you. Help us cast out negative thoughts causing us to worry or making us feel undeserving or jealous. Give us courage to ask for forgiveness from anyone we've envied or judged. There's comfort in knowing you made each of us individual and unique and we're on our own earthly journey. Please keep our ears listening to your still, small voice. Amen.

HUSBANDS AND WIVES GRIEVE DIFFERENTLY

I'm sure Toby is grieving in his own way, but I wanted to see him cry too for the child we may never have. Instead he comforted me as I cried into his chest each night. —Kim

"WHY ARE YOU CRYING, HANNAH?" ELKANAH WOULD ASK. "WHY AREN'T YOU EATING? WHY BE DOWNHEARTED JUST BECAUSE YOU HAVE NO CHILDREN? YOU HAVE ME—ISN'T THAT BETTER THAN HAVING TEN SONS?"
—1 Samuel 1:8 NLT

Shannon's Journal

Dear God,

Infertility is hard on marriage because it makes you question everything in life. In our support group, they had us write down date night ideas and favorite things we did before we were married. That was helpful.

A lot of the focus during treatments is on me, like I carry more of the pressure than Dan. I immerse in it in a way he doesn't. Dan thinks about it for the appointment or the procedure, and then he's able to leave it, almost as if he can compartmentalize and separate it from other things in his life. And thank you that he can, because he's there to give me much-needed perspective on the situation, but sometimes it also leaves me feeling misunderstood and alone. At times, one of us is willing to go further with alternatives than the other is ready to consider.

It's hard trying to work out all this in the midst of grief that follows you daily. We don't make the best decisions when we're grieving, and we don't always treat each other the best, either.

Grieving together, Shannon

A Mommy-in-Waiting Shares

My husband Tim and I struggled with infertility for four and a half years with two surgeries for endometriosis, invasive tests, procedures, and an unsuccessful IVF attempt. The specialist told us we couldn't have children, so we decided to adopt.

Two weeks before our adoption interview, we were pregnant. At the thirty-eight week appointment, the OB had trouble finding a heartbeat and, after an emergency C-section, there was no heartbeat. By the time they got Mikayla's heart beating, she was in liver and kidney failure with no brain function. We were on the same heartbreaking page agreeing to remove her from life support. The hardest thing I've ever done is physically letting go of my little girl. It's amazing what God gives you the strength to do. Mikayla, "gift from God," is an organ donor, and she let us know we could get pregnant, which we successfully did twice through embryo adoption and naturally.

Men and women process grief so differently; we have to adjust our expectations of each other. Tim doesn't understand my need to emotionally connect with Mikayla on her birthday by going to the cemetery, and I don't understand him not wanting to be there because it brings up bad memories. We're starting to understand we have different needs, different ways of coping, and that's OK. It hasn't always been that way, but God is growing us. —Sarah

A Daddy-in-Waiting Shares

When a routine ultrasound showed our baby had hydrocephalus, a cleft palate, and a right hand that couldn't open, Tiff and I went home and wept. We asked many from the church to pray, and we named him Ezekiel, "God's strength." People loved Ezekiel and loved us by praying for healing but, above all, that God's will be done. Then God revealed his will and our answer to prayer in a way we didn't want. God took Ezekiel home. Our sad cries of "Why? Why? Why?" will likely never be answered. How could there be an answer sufficient to us?

I think if we hadn't gone through infertility, losing Ezekiel would have been even more difficult. It's by no means easy, but that road of infertility we walked down, and continue to walk, made it easier. We already knew loss, and we knew our different ways of communicating, looking at things, and responding to situations. That knowledge, along with our faith in God, has helped us stay close to each other, instead of drawing us apart, through this tremendous loss. —Simon

Janet's Mentoring Moment

Many of us marry our exact opposite, which is beneficial in a crisis when one panics while the other ponders. However, differences can also lead to conflict, hurt feelings, and misunderstandings. You may want your spouse to feel as badly as you do, and when it appears he or she doesn't, you assume he or she doesn't care. Those presumptions are counterproductive and unfair. Try viewing different response styles as a gift. Thank God that one of you stays calm while the other indulges in the luxury of falling apart.

In his article "When Mr. Fix-It Won't Do," Bob Perry wrote about lessons he learned from his wife's miscarriage:

A husband can't fully understand a wife's instantaneous emotional attachment toward a newly conceived child for which he feels a detached loss for someone he never knew. A husband can't make the pain go away or understand the length of time his wife clings to grief. A husband needs to show his grief; it helps his wife realize she isn't alone and it may help her overcome feelings of anger or despair. A husband can't fix this but he can support, encourage, and love his wife fully.[1]

You both are grieving the loss of your original dream of how you would become parents, and one may be feeling personally responsible or in a darker place than the other. Choose to let the infertility struggle draw you closer together as you comfort and love each other.

God's Love Letter to You

Dear_____ and_____,

To comfort all who mourn and provide for those who grieve, I will bestow on them a crown of beauty instead of ashes, the oil of gladness instead of mourning, and a garment of praise instead of a spirit of despair. They will be called oaks of righteousness, a planting of the Lord for the display of my splendor (Isa. 61:2–3, paraphrased).

Grieving with you, God

Couple's Prayer

Lord, We do grieve differently. Please help us understand and support each other. Don't let us fall apart at the same time so we can lift the other one up out of the mire of grief. Give us your vision for our family. Remind us that you put the two of us together for better or worse, even though "worse" seems unbearable. We need to see the rainbow at the end of our dark storm. Help us focus on our love and not our loss. Amen.

ALLOWING YOURSELF TO MOURN

I grieved for the embryos that never implanted. I knew them as our babies regardless of how far they had developed. —Melanie

My heart was broken, and I was mourning the death of my hopes, my dreams, and my babies. —Danette

JOB STOOD UP AND TORE HIS ROBE IN GRIEF. THEN HE SHAVED HIS HEAD AND FELL TO THE GROUND BEFORE GOD.
—Job 1:20 NLT

Kim's Journal

Dear God,

We're closing the door on trying to get pregnant and walking through the door we feel you're opening for us to adopt. Every agency I contact tells me the same thing: to prepare for adoption, we must come to terms with possibly never having a baby biologically. Many days I'm excited about adopting; other days I cry about not being able to conceive on my own.

I have the same feelings as when we were doing artificial insemination—excitement at the possibilities, yet grieving that it takes so much work trying to get there. The shots, brown paper bags, and numerous doctors' appointments definitely wasn't the romantic way I envisioned having a child with the love of my life; now with adoption, there's endless paperwork, interviews, classes, home inspections, and waiting. I won't get to experience hearing the first heartbeat, feeling the first kick, watching my body change, wearing maternity clothes, or nursing—providing nutrients and a special bond between my baby and me.

Coming to terms with the losses is painful. The adoption agency we've selected instructed us in the importance of acknowledging our feelings and the pain associated with them *before* we can move on. If we continue holding on to the hope and dream of having our own baby, we won't be fully open to adoption.

God, I realize being a parent isn't about being pregnant—that's my own selfish desire—it's about loving, nurturing, protecting, teaching, and preparing a child to know and love you. It's not about me. You have a plan, and your plan always is good if we just trust in you. When we accept this, we'll be able to move beyond what we're missing out on and look forward to new experiences. Adoption isn't our last resort at becoming parents. We want a child. You, God, have spoken clearly that we're to go this direction. If we just let go and let you work, you will fulfill our dreams of being parents.

Expectantly mourning, Kim

Two Mommies-in-Waiting Share

Before we pursued adoptive parenthood, Robert and I allowed ourselves to mourn the death of our dream for biological parenthood. Our grieving was private. Few people offered condolences. There was no memorial service . . . no one to mourn. We grieved the loss of babies who never existed—of babies who would never exist.

Robert and I made the transition quickly, replacing the dashed hopes infertility wrought with high hopes to adopt. But I still experienced occasional twinges of longing for a birth child. When I saw pregnant women, jolts of jealousy coursed through me. When friends discussed childbirth, a shadow of sadness crept over me. I had assumed that my commitment to building a family through adoption would put those feelings to rest. I had assumed we had resolved our infertility.

Then it hit me. Infertility is a chronic medical condition, one that requires management over the course of a lifetime. I needed to focus less on *resolving* my infertility and more on *managing* it. Managing infertility means admitting it wounds me—physically, emotionally, and spiritually. Managing infertility means I can expect old wounds to rip open when I attend baby showers or watch a mother nurse her child. Managing infertility means allowing myself to wonder what it would be like to have a child with Robert's blue eyes and my thick hair; a child who mimics Robert's habit of misplacing keys or my obsession with cleaning house when I'm stressed. Managing infertility means accepting the fact that, while my desire for a birth child has diminished, it never will entirely disappear.[2]
—Laura Christianson

We're hoping to get to the place where we can consider adoption again. We first need to deal with the grief of infertility. We don't want to view adoption as a Band-Aid—a substitution for what we couldn't have—or hold an adopted child to an ideological, unreasonable standard of a biological child we never had. We'd also love our relationship, and our individual relationships with God, to heal from the stresses of infertility. —Mel

Janet's Mentoring Moment
Infertility is fraught with volatile emotions of loss. Some couples incur the tangible, heart-wrenching loss of miscarriages or stillborns, but all infertile couples experience the less tangible loss of a dream: an easy, unassisted, "natural" pregnancy resulting in children who have traits from both of your families.

You may also be grieving your image of God and the role you thought he would play in your life. You're angry with him for letting infertility happen to you. Anything buried alive has energy, which eventually erupts explosively, and that's what happens to unresolved feelings. Job understood this concept when he said, "Even if I say, 'I'll put all this behind me, I'll look on the bright side and force a smile,' all these troubles would still be like grit in my gut" (Job 9:27–28 *The Message*).

The losses you're mourning will take time to work through, so allow yourself to grieve completely, and then make a conscious decision to move on in the way you feel God is leading you as a couple. In *The One Year Walk with God Devotional*, Chris Tiegreen reminds us that, "In the midst of our pain, God speaks promises. In the far reaches of our grief, He reaches even farther. He promises comfort to those who know the grief of this world. He offers Himself in comfort."[3]

God's Love Letter to You

Dear_____ and_____,
Blessed are those who mourn, for they will be comforted (Matt. 5:4).
Your comforter, God

Couple's Prayer

Oh Jesus, This is such a sad and difficult journey, and we could never make it without your love and support. When will the mourning end? When will we wake up and be happy to see a new day? Hold us, Lord. We need our mourning turned to dancing again, soon. Amen.

THE GRIEVING PROCESS

The doctor informed us it wasn't a viable pregnancy; the "egg" hadn't developed. Our hearts were broken. It didn't feel like an "undeveloped egg," but the loss of a baby, the loss of a dream. —Michele

Tricking myself with false hope, EPT after EPT, always with the same negative response, I am pained beyond grief. —Robin

WHEN RACHEL SAW THAT SHE WAS NOT BEARING JACOB ANY CHILDREN,
SHE BECAME JEALOUS OF HER SISTER. SO SHE SAID TO JACOB,
"GIVE ME CHILDREN, OR I'LL DIE!"
—Genesis 30:1

Kim's Journal

Dear God,
Receiving the invitation to Shannon's baby shower was a reminder that, as I'd been making my way through endless adoption paperwork and lists of things to do, Shannon was experiencing pregnancy. Rationally, I knew I would have a baby too someday, but I couldn't grasp the reality. I could use distance as an excuse not to attend, but I wasn't working and had plenty of free

time. My mom told me it would mean a lot to Shannon for me to come, but being festive and joyful was going to take more than I had in me, not to mention seeing her visibly pregnant.

With a lot of prayer and persuasion from my mom, I decided to attend. The day of the shower I had an upset stomach and was tired, but for Shannon's sake, I put on my happy face. I didn't want her to see me feeling sorry for myself or have the spotlight on me.

With a forced smile, I did all right through the games and festivities until gift opening. Shannon emotionally thanked everyone for coming and for their support and prayers through her struggles getting pregnant. Then she shared what a miracle this baby was . . . I didn't hear the rest as I ran out to the backyard sobbing, and my mom followed. We sat hugging and crying.

I couldn't pretend happiness any longer. I wanted to make that speech thanking everyone for their prayers and thanking God for the miracle baby growing inside me. Why couldn't I have that, too? Why didn't you, God, let us both get pregnant together? Why would you do this *only* to me? Aside from my pain, I felt horrible listening to Shannon: I didn't deserve her thanks. I hadn't prayed for her, and I hadn't been supportive either. Selfishly, I had only prayed for myself.

This was a revelation: What if it had been the other way around, and this was my shower, and Shannon was sitting in the back of the room wishing she could be in my shoes? Would I want her being resentful and bitter toward me? Shannon's baby was coming, so I needed to get a grip and be happy for her. What was happening to me wasn't her fault. I would no longer hold her accountable for my pain. I needed to stop letting this eat me up inside and release her. My bitterness wasn't fair to either of us.

Working through the grieving process, Kim

Two Mommies-in-Waiting Share

Over time, I had an arsenal of TTC gear: a mini microscope for saliva, a bathroom strewn with OPKs and EPTs, multiple basal body thermometers, expensive herbs and vitamins, and empty Clomid bottles. I lost count of the number of cycles we consciously tried to conceive. I was prayed over and many prayed for us.

Around year six, after a long bout of hyper-TTC, my emotions and attitude plummeted. I spent years in an infertility-rooted depression. There were moments I thought dying would be better; life didn't seem worth living without children. I couldn't bear the death of my life dream. Perhaps a different spouse would increase my chances of being a mom? Maybe a younger spouse with an affluent career could make adoption a reality? Yes, I considered divorce, an affair, and going against my husband by ordering from a sperm bank.

Thank God, I didn't act on those unrighteous ideas, but I hit such a low I ended up on Prozac spending most days in bed. The depression didn't begin to subside until I faced my error of making a baby more important than anything and everyone, and I stopped my life from orbiting around the golden baby idol. There still are moments of sadness, reminiscing about what could have been, followed by a healthy cry. I spent over a decade yearning for children; those dreams always will be in my memory, with an ambiguous sense of loss. —Rachel L.

I began taking a mild antidepressant that helped the physical symptoms, but I needed to deal with the raw emotions from infertility. I was overtaken by anxiety and fighting to get my life back. It was a long, difficult process requiring lots of hard, necessary work. I went to a counselor who specialized in infertility issues and also was infertile. Talking to someone with my same experiences and releasing the years of built-up emotions was therapeutic. Not being chosen by birthparents during this time was a blessing in disguise. —Sharon

Janet's Mentoring Moment

Grief accompanies infertility as pain, suffering, and loss plague your mind and heart. You're not showing a lack of faith to experience grief. Christ grieved. "He began to be filled with anguish and deep distress. He told them, 'My soul is crushed with grief to the point of death'" (Matt. 26:38 NLT).

On page 267 in the Sanity Tools, you'll find the Stages of Grief. Acknowledge where you are in the grieving process, and allow yourself time to work through each step. Both of you may progress at a different pace, but it's critical to keep moving. Some women, like the biblical Rachel and the Mommies-in-Waiting above, stay stuck at the depression stage and become dangerously desperate. Gay Lynne wrote, "My life seemed to come to an end when my husband Dan said he would be 'OK' without kids. I became very angry with God, and very angry with my husband. That's when I became suicidal. Would life be worth living without the one thing I always had so greatly desired?"

The answer is yes. Life is worth living, as Rachel L. discovered when she realized she was valuing having a child more than she valued even God. Whatever you think about most becomes your god—your idol—and thus begins a deterioration of your relationship with God, who says, "You must not have any other god but me" (Exod. 20:3 NLT). Righting your relationship with God is the first step in overcoming the brokenness of depression and desperation.

In your deepest, darkest times, you don't think rationally. Look at the Signs of Depression, and Sharon's symptoms on page 268. If you're experiencing any of these symptoms, seek help from your doctor and church. Sharon and Rachel L. took medication, but both realized an important truth: while medication might help the physical symptoms, they needed to deal with the emotional and spiritual issues.

Michele found solace in the Christian support group Mommies Enduring Neonatal Death (M.E.N.D., see page 252). "I no longer felt so alone, and my faith was renewed," she said. Check to see if your church, or a church near you, has a grief support group. There also may be one at a nearby hospital or fertility clinic.

If attending baby showers is too painful, don't force yourself. Or tell the hostess you'll be arriving late and leaving early, or take someone with you for moral support. When the shower is for a family member, remember you are related to this new little life. As Kim learned, you must progressively transition through the grief process so you don't lose hope and become bitter, cynical, and discouraged.

God's Love Letter to You

Dear_____ and_____,

Go ahead and be angry. You do well to be angry—but don't use your anger as fuel for revenge. And don't stay angry. Don't go to bed angry. Don't give the Devil that kind of foothold in your life (Eph. 4:26–27 *The Message*). Don't be afraid, for I am with you. Do not be discouraged, for I am your God. I will strengthen you and help you. I will hold you up with my victorious right hand (Isa. 41:10 NLT).

Your strength, God

Couple's Prayer

Merciful God, We cried out to you. O Lord, we begged you for mercy. . . . Hear us, Lord, and have mercy on us. Help us, O Lord. You have turned our mourning into joyful dancing. You have taken away our clothes of mourning and clothed us with joy, that we might sing praises to you and not be silent. O Lord our God, we will give you thanks forever! Amen (Ps. 30:8–12 NLT, paraphrased).

Your Letter to God

Part of the healing process of mourning is putting your feelings down on paper. Pour out your heart to God. Feel the release with each written word describing the emotions holding you captive. Let the refreshing balm of Jesus' love wash over you.

Dear God,   *Date:*

_____

_____

_____

_____

_____

_____

_____

_____

_____

_____

_____

_____

_____

_____

_____

_____

_____

_____

Chapter Fifteen

DISCOVERING A NEW FOCUS AND PURPOSE

I'M NOT SAYING THAT I HAVE THIS ALL TOGETHER, THAT I HAVE IT MADE.
BUT I AM WELL ON MY WAY, REACHING OUT FOR CHRIST,
WHO HAS SO WONDROUSLY REACHED OUT FOR ME.
FRIENDS, DON'T GET ME WRONG: BY NO MEANS DO I
COUNT MYSELF AN EXPERT IN ALL OF THIS,
BUT I'VE GOT MY EYE ON THE GOAL, WHERE GOD
IS BECKONING US ONWARD—TO JESUS.
I'M OFF AND RUNNING, AND I'M NOT TURNING BACK.
SO LET'S KEEP FOCUSED ON THAT GOAL, THOSE OF US
WHO WANT EVERYTHING GOD HAS FOR US.
IF ANY OF YOU HAVE SOMETHING ELSE IN MIND, SOME-
THING LESS THAN TOTAL COMMITMENT,
GOD WILL CLEAR YOUR BLURRED VISION—YOU'LL SEE IT YET!
NOW THAT WE'RE ON THE RIGHT TRACK, LET'S STAY ON IT.
STICK WITH ME, FRIENDS.
KEEP TRACK OF THOSE YOU SEE RUNNING THIS SAME
COURSE, HEADED FOR THIS SAME GOAL.
—Philippians 3:12–17 *The Message*

Finding Purpose in Your Infertility

We feel that because God allowed us to experience infertility, he must have a child out there, born or unborn, waiting for us to call our own. —Tiffany and Simon

I CRY OUT TO GOD MOST HIGH, TO GOD WHO WILL FULFILL HIS PURPOSE FOR ME.
—Psalm 57:2 NLT

Kim's Journal

Dear God,

One weekend at church, the guest speaker was Bruce Wilkinson, author of *The Dream Giver*. He taught that you, the Dream Giver, give everyone a "Big Dream" which can change lives.

Obstacles to achieving that Big Dream might actually be a series of opportunities guiding toward our destiny. We may have to leave our comfort zone to pursue our dream.

He told the tragic story of seeing an orphan boy dead from hunger and exposure on a sidewalk in Africa. He sadly thought that God had given someone the dream to take care of that orphan, but the person hadn't fulfilled his or her dream. God, I sat there with a lump in my throat. It's like the speaker was talking directly to me. I thought: *My all-encompassing dream was to be a mother, and all I've hit are roadblocks. What are you trying to tell me, God? Is your dream for me to adopt a child? Is that why you've closed my womb?* Shivers ran up and down my spine, as I finally came to realize what your plan might be for us.

Apparently the speaker only told that story at our service! I shivered again at the thought that you had placed us in that service to hear that specific story, while in other services people heard different stories about their specific dreams. God, you *are* talking to me. I can hear you now clearly. I feel your comforting, assuring presence. You always will be there for me. I need to have patience and trust that you won't abandon me. You will fulfill my deepest desire. Maybe adoption is your plan after all. Maybe a child out there is meant for us.

Finding purpose, Kim

A Mommy-in-Waiting Shares

I knew our not being able to conceive biologically didn't mean we couldn't be parents. I felt that in five years, God would have two beautiful children in our home, handpicked for us for his purpose. I told all who would listen: Don't feel sorry for me. God has a plan and a purpose for our infertility. It's in Jeremiah 29:11–13, my favorite verses I hold on to each day. This is not to say there weren't hard and difficult days. —Karen

Janet's Mentoring Moment

Karen had heard God clearly. She and her husband Ken adopted frozen embryos through the Snowflakes program and got pregnant with twin girls, but one was stillborn. Ken said in the eulogy for their lost Carissa: "A baby is a gift, a new entity, a precious individual soul loved by God. We are created for a purpose; there is a reason for our being here. In her short life Carissa made us realize that we cannot control or predict the future; she made us rely on God. She even helped her stubborn dad finish his quest for faith and now I *know* I'll get to see her again."

What a tremendous witness to friends and family for Karen and Ken to find purpose in their tragedy and use it to glorify God. Instead of rejecting God, Ken found God and eternal life.

Everyone is searching for purpose in the circumstances of life, and we'll never fully understand everything this side of heaven. God didn't purposely cause your infertility and loss, but he can use it for a good purpose. God never wastes a hurt. His plans are for good, not for harm. God brings the best out of the worst circumstances—maybe it's the softening of a heart with deeper compassion, a different perspective or reevaluation of priorities, a new or closer walk with him, or a new ministry. Bruce Wilkinson writes:

> Why did that nameless boy die on the sidewalk? I believe his Need was someone else's Dream—a Big important Dream that had not been embraced and pursued. That's a sobering conclusion, I know. Yet it certainly cannot be God's will that any child die alone and abandoned. Surely God placed a particular set of interests and abilities in one person, somewhere in this world, and put that person in a time and place where Great Things could happen—*should* have happened—for that boy. Will you take up the challenge that so many have avoided?[1]

God's Love Letter to You
*Dear*_____*and*_____,
My purpose is to give life in all its fullness (John 10:10 NLT).
Your Lord and Savior, Jesus Christ

Couple's Prayer
Our loving Lord and Father of our Savior, Jesus Christ, We look at this Son and see the God who cannot be seen. We look at this Son and see God's original purpose in everything created. For everything, absolutely everything, above and below, visible and invisible, and rank after rank after rank of angels—everything got started in him and finds its purpose in him. He was there before any of it came into existence and holds it all together right up to this moment. Amen. (Col. 1:15–17 *The Message,* paraphrased)

CHANGING FOCUS

We continue to cycle through emotions; however, time has softened the degree to which we experience difficult feelings. Primarily, we have begun to accept our situation and are learning and open to making the most of the options still available to us. —Tiffany and Simon

HERE'S WHAT I WANT YOU TO DO: FIND A QUIET, SECLUDED PLACE SO YOU WON'T BE TEMPTED TO ROLE-PLAY BEFORE GOD. JUST BE THERE AS SIMPLY AND HONESTLY AS YOU CAN MANAGE. THE FOCUS WILL SHIFT FROM YOU TO GOD, AND YOU WILL BEGIN TO SENSE HIS GRACE.
—Matthew 6:6 *The Message*

Kim's Journal

Dear God,

Changing our focus toward adoption, I started researching adoption agencies online. I came across a program called Snowflakes that helps couples with unused IVF frozen embryos place their precious unborn babies up for adoption so they aren't destroyed or used for science. If we chose this path, the adopted embryos would be implanted in me, and I would carry the pregnancy to term.

Wow! I had never heard of this. I actually could have an opportunity to experience pregnancy, labor, and breastfeeding. My blood would run through this child's veins as he or she grew inside me, so there would be that connection as well. We wouldn't be creating life but giving an opportunity for a previously created life. What an awesome thought!

With the increased numbers of couples choosing IVF, there are hundreds of thousands of frozen embryos without a home. I had such respect for parents choosing to donate their unborn babies as a gift to infertile couples. What a loving and responsible thing to do.

This sounded exciting, so we prayed about it. For reasons we didn't understand, we felt called to go another direction, but I always thought this was such a wonderful ministry to give the gift of life a chance at life.

Changing focus, Kim

A Mommy-in-Waiting Shares

I let go of my dreams—not my hopes, but the plans I had for myself. I released God to work *his* dreams and plans for me. I felt an incredible peace and strength, and for the first time, Jeff and I could talk openly about our desires for babies and the struggle we were facing not having them. We felt God's go-ahead for testing to bring closure to this chapter of our journey. The specialist delivered expected news: "I'm so sorry; I really wanted to get this one, but unfortunately you cannot have children." We were sad but not surprised: it wasn't a shock, but a confirmation that gave us permission to move on in another direction.

We thought the only other option in building a family was adoption. As we changed our focus, this excited and terrified us. The Lord gave me a Scripture I claimed as my promise from him, and it became my prayer. Psalm 113:9 says, "He settles the barren woman in her home as a happy mother of children. Praise the LORD." Jeff and I didn't know when, but we felt the Lord's confirmation that someday we would be parents. In the meantime, we got the word out to family members and close friends that we were thinking and praying about adoption.
—Danette

Janet's Mentoring Moment

Infertility often requires a change in focus and a reassessment of goals. Acknowledging your primary goal helps bring priorities into focus. Some of the couples sharing their stories felt adopting frozen embryos through the Snowflakes program or a private attorney was the best of both worlds—experiencing pregnancy and adoption. Their change in focus from trying to procreate to co-create also resulted in a ministry of providing the opportunity of life to a life waiting to be born. The couples who donated their frozen embryos changed their focus from trying to create life to giving life to their creations and blessing another infertile couple with a chance to experience pregnancy and give brith to a child.

Several couples changed their focus from trying to have a child to adopting, and others decided to remain childless and serve the wider community and family of God.

Heidi Schlumpf in her article "Inconceivable" suggests that "Being able to experience new life—whether through a successful pregnancy, adoption, [embryo adoption or donation], or choosing to remain childless and focusing on serving the wider community—after the 'death' of infertility mirrors the resurrection and redemption. Although the pain is real, ultimately many couples find their faith helps them move through the grief to make life-giving choices for themselves and for others."[2]

Wherever your heart is leading you and whatever path to parenthood you're pursuing or have chosen to stop pursuing, keep your eyes on Jesus—he will bring everything into focus for you.

God's Love Letter to You

Dear_____ and_____ ,

If you are humble, I will lead you in what is right and teach you my ways. If you keep my covenant and obey my decrees I, the Lord, will lead you with unfailing love and faithfulness (Ps. 25:9–10 NLT, paraphrased).

Your refocus, God

Couple's Prayer

Lord, It isn't easy changing our mind and our plans. We thought we knew exactly how we were going to become parents, and all those doors are closing. Father, give us an open mind and an open heart to see the doors you are opening to take us in a different direction. Help us keep our focus on you and not on ourselves and our circumstances. Amen.

HOW CAN GOD USE YOUR INFERTILITY?

God's plan is the best, and we're living best when we're totally, even blindly, surrendered to his will. There is purpose in all pain. Being grateful in the midst of it allows for a peaceful journey. —Robin

THE LORD HAS A REASON FOR EVERYTHING HE DOES.
—Proverbs 16:4 CEV

Kim's Journal

Dear God,

As I continued researching how you might want to use us and also fulfill our dream to be parents, I came across Bethany Christian Services, an adoption agency. They specialize in helping infertile Christian couples adopt a child through an open adoption, either domestically or internationally. I contacted their office, and they invited us to attend an adoption orientation meeting. I had so many questions and was so excited to hear about their program; I could hardly wait.

You haven't deserted me. You love me and have a greater plan than I ever could imagine. This isn't just about me anymore. It's so much bigger. Adoption is supposed to be our ministry. We're going to adopt a baby!

Moving on, Kim

A Mommy-in-Waiting Shares

I experienced infertility twenty years ago. I had three miscarriages when I was in my twenties and had to have a hysterectomy at age thirty-five. It was emotionally painful, but I learned about God's love and sovereignty in my life. I learned God is the One who opens and closes the womb, and he has a purpose for everything he does. I'm now forty-six and very content as a childless Christian woman and wife. Fulfilling my desire to help children, I recently was working as a tutor with elementary-age children in an area with extreme poverty and homelessness. I have many Christian friends who, like myself, weren't able to bear children, but with God's grace lead full and productive lives. —Linda

Janet's Mentoring Moment

Once you accept that God has a purpose and you're agreeable to changing your focus, if necessary, the next step is to stay in tune with God to learn what, where, and how he *will* use your infertility to further his earthly work. When you're ready, he *will* reveal his plan that fits your personality, talents, gifts, and environment. He *will* fulfill his purpose and plan in your life if you let him.

When Kim and Toby decided becoming parents was their primary purpose, God helped them view adoption as a ministry: providing a loving home for a child in need. When their focus changed, so did their hearts. They realized as Christians we're all adopted into the family of God. Ephesians 1:5 (NLT) took on new meaning to them: "God decided in advance to adopt us into his own family by bringing us to himself through Jesus Christ."

Bruce Wilkinson writes, "Your Dream is meant to be about more than itself or you. A God-given Dream brings you together with what God wants to do in His world *through you*."[3]

God's Love Letter to You

Dear_____ and_____,

Give yourselves to me. Surrender your whole being to me to be used for righteous purposes (Rom. 6:14 GNT, paraphrased).

I will use you, God

Couple's Prayer

Heavenly Father, Help us see our infertility as a ministry to be used for your purpose. You are a purposeful God. Your promise has been tested through and through, and we, your servants, love it dearly. Your righteousness is eternally right, your revelation is the only truth. Even though troubles came down on us hard, your commands always gave us delight. The way you tell us to live is always right; help us understand it so we can live to the fullest. We call out at the top of our lungs, "God! Answer! We'll do whatever you say." We called to you, "Save us so we can carry out all your instructions." Amen. (Ps. 119:140–146 *The Message,* paraphrased)

Your Letter to God

Have you looked for God's purpose in your journey? If not, ask him now to reveal how he can be glorified and how he wants to use you. If you've seen glimpses of his purpose, write them down so you don't forget, and ask him to continue the revelations.

Dear God,   *Date:*

_____

_____

_____

_____

_____

_____

_____

_____

_____

_____

_____

_____

_____

Chapter Sixteen

SECONDARY INFERTILITY

WILL THE LORD WALK OFF AND LEAVE US FOR GOOD?
WILL HE NEVER SMILE AGAIN?
IS HIS LOVE WORN THREADBARE?
HAS HIS SALVATION PROMISE BURNED OUT?
HAS GOD FORGOTTEN HIS MANNERS?
HAS HE ANGRILY STALKED OFF AND LEFT US?
"JUST MY LUCK," I SAID. "THE HIGH GOD GOES OUT OF BUSINESS
JUST THE MOMENT I NEED HIM."
ONCE AGAIN I'LL GO OVER WHAT GOD HAS DONE,
LAY OUT ON THE TABLE THE ANCIENT WONDERS;
I'LL PONDER ALL THE THINGS YOU'VE ACCOMPLISHED,
AND GIVE A LONG, LOVING LOOK AT YOUR ACTS.
—Psalm 77:7–12 *The Message*

We're Ready for Another Baby

My miracle son is ten, and we've since prayed for and tried unsuccessfully to have more children. God is for me, and he knows what's best for me, even when it doesn't make sense to my human mind. Some things I'll understand later in this life, and some I'll have to wait to understand until I see him face to face. —Tressia

I HAVE LEARNED TO BE CONTENT WHATEVER THE CIRCUMSTANCES.
—Philippians 4:11

Shannon's Journal

Dear God,
I really enjoyed my pregnancy with Josh and felt great. Labor and birth didn't go so easy. Honestly, I think I labored for twenty-three hours because I was afraid to be a mom. I didn't

know if I had it in me . . . the patience, love, sleep depravation. Well, I learned to love my baby, and my love has grown each day since his birth.

Two years later, when Dan and I decided we were ready for a second child, we expected IVF to be successful with the first transfer, like it was with Josh. So we scheduled a time to go through the process again with our frozen embryos. Lord, we were hopeful when one attached and so sad when, seven weeks later, I miscarried. Well, the embryos were frozen and not as viable, so we'll save up our money and try again. You know how badly we want a brother or sister for Joshua. It looks like it might take a couple of tries this time, so we better get started. I know our turn is coming.

Like I told my friend Stephanie when she was discouraged and I gave her hope with the miracle story of Josh, "It only takes one good one." I always saw the best for her. I still have the cross she sent me with the word "Believe," and when I see that cross, I say a prayer for my next child and thank you for Stephanie's baby girl.

Longing for another child, Shannon

A Mommy-in-Waiting Shares

When our daughter Dana was a year old, my husband and I were ready for another child. Since I got pregnant quickly the first time, we expected a second child right on schedule. When I didn't become pregnant, we consulted a doctor.

I began praying God's promises in Scripture. I reminded him of Jeremiah 29:11 promising me hope and a future; Psalm 37:4 says if I delight in him, he'll give me the desires of my heart; and Psalm 84:11 (NASB) says, "No good thing does He withhold from those who walk uprightly." Then I realized God's promises didn't mean he was promising me another baby.

I spent the next soul-searching days in prayer, and God reminded me of my longtime desire to write encouraging books for women, but life as a young mother got too hectic. I told the Lord I still wanted to write, even if it meant not having another baby. I surrendered my desire to have a second child. Several days later, the doctor called with fertility test results: "You know that miracle baby you've been praying for? You already had her, three years ago!" My husband and I had fertility incompatibility and shouldn't have been able to have *any* children!

I had been given my promised blessing. I'm thankful for God's plans, not my own. And I'm thankful I was ready to receive his news as a blessing, rather than with bitterness. The second child has never come, but I've published ten books and have a speaking ministry to women. My husband and I realize God's goodness in knowing what we could handle—financially, emotionally, and otherwise—in giving us only one child. —Cindi McMenamin

Janet's Mentoring Moment

Cindi made a great discovery: our plans and ideas of what is "good" don't always align with God's good plans. Through prayer and reading her Bible, God brought Cindi to the place of accepting that he had fulfilled his promises, and now it was time for her to do the Lord's work. Ministry might not be God's plan for you, but he does have a plan, and he will reveal it to you when you spend time with him.

And spend time with the child you have. While you're longing to give your child a sibling, what your child really wants is you—*loving*, not *longing*, parents. Be careful not to shift all your emotions and efforts to creating another child and lose sight of God's creation in your arms.

God's Love Letter to You

Dear_____ and_____,
You have left the love you had in the beginning. So remember where you were before you fell. Change your hearts and do what you did at first (Rev. 2:4–5 NCV).
Your first love, Jesus Christ

A Couple's Prayer

Lord, Please help us be content with the many blessings you have given us and the precious child you have already brought into our lives. Help us learn to savor what we have and not dwell on what we don't have. If it isn't your plan for us to have another child, please remove this gnawing desire in our souls. If your plan is to expand our family, please give us perseverance and patience and show us how to fulfill that dream. Amen.

WHY ISN'T IT WORKING?

God, are you listening? If you don't want us to have another child, please take away my desire for one. —Alice

How long, O Lord? Will you forget me forever?
How long will you hide your face from me?
How long must I wrestle with my thoughts and
every day have sorrow in my heart?
—Psalm 13:1–2

Shannon's Journal

Dear God,

Here I am writing of another miscarriage at nine weeks. I haven't wanted to write. Not this time. At times the pain is too much. Too much to cry, to write, to do anything. I've listened to a lot of music that warms my heavy, hurting heart. God, I can accept it wasn't my time, but will it ever be? I've invested a lot and it hurts. We had just started to get excited. It's taken a toll. The reality of the loss is too painful to face every day. I can only take it in bits and pieces. I can only cry on occasions. I purposely put it out of my mind.

I see all these people around me having more children. I'm jealous. I'm envious. It's hard being around them. I feel bad saying this, but I feel no happiness for them, only sadness. I feel like weeping. I don't want to hold their babies; I want to hold mine. If I do hold them, I can only do it for a short time. It's painful to hear their laughs and cries. I got angry today. Are you shutting the door to being a mother again?

I just want to shop and clean and clean some more or paint. After I'm done, the hurt's still there. Like it's waiting for me to visit and give it time to do its work, but I can't—not yet. Sometimes, I just sit feeling frozen. I can't think straight, and I'm not motivated to get up and do anything. This goes in cycles: I feel fine, the next day I'm back to square one, crying again. I'm less patient and more irritable lately. It seems I'm angry at everybody and everything.

God, I don't know what to do. I really want another child. I feel desperate. I'm frustrated. You give such good gifts . . . you've walked me through so much, but I have no perspective. I can't see the big picture. I don't feel at peace with adopting, yet I want a child like yesterday. I think about it all the time. Calm my mind, my thoughts . . . give me your peace. I'm so torn up inside. I feel impatient . . . unsettled about my family being incomplete.

Feeling incomplete, Shannon

A Mommy-in-Waiting Shares

Our hearts felt the pain listening to our son Evan pray, "Dear Jesus, please bring me a baby brother or sister. Amen." My pregnancy with Evan was normal. When I became pregnant a year later, our son was stillborn at twenty-two weeks. We were devastated and wondered if God would ever give us another child. I had four more pregnancies in four years—all ending by the fourteenth week. My physical, spiritual, and emotional states were up and down. It was exhausting. Some days, it was all I could do to remember God is love and keep breathing. I was tired of anticipating a birth, creating milk for a baby who would never taste it, and then leaving the hospital with empty arms.

As I grieved the loss of each child, within the depths of my heart a glimmer of hope remained that I would someday carry a baby to full term, and I clung to Jeremiah 29:11. After the last miscarriage, God gave us Isaiah 43:18–19, which we took as encouragement to pursue adoption, and God started opening doors. We no longer felt his silence after praying, but after a year of waiting for word from a state adoption agency, we still were no closer to having a baby.

Finally, we shared our deepest struggles with a close friend who introduced us to private adoption facilitators that bring families and birth parents together. A few weeks later, we selected birth parents meeting our requirements, who felt unable to provide for their child and were considering an abortion. Thirteen hours after her birth, we introduced our daughter to the big brother who had prayed for her. We're so thankful and feel like a complete family. God has even taken away my desire for more children. —Alice

Janet's Mentoring Moment

Mommy-in-Waiting Melanie finally had a second pregnancy with twins through IVF, but one of the twins died before birth. Melanie had a vision that might be helpful if you've experienced such a devastating loss: "I had the hope of seeing our baby again. I had a vision of him sitting on Jesus' lap in safety, in love, and without having experienced the sadness of this world. This loss was significant and we grieved tremendously, but the time I had spent with the Lord prepared me."

Verna suffered one miscarriage before her first child and four during unsuccessful attempts to have a second child. She confirmed the importance of spending time with the Lord during this trying and sad time. "I felt like God was telling me to stop focusing on myself and my wants for another child and read my Bible. Stop trying to control where we were headed and instead follow God." Even when you don't see God at work, he's working on your heart and your future.

God's Love Letter to You

Dear_____ and_____,

Forget the former things; do not dwell on the past. See, I am doing a new thing! Now it springs up; do you not perceive it? I am making a way in the desert and streams in the wasteland (Isa. 43:18–19).

I haven't forgotten you, God

Couple's Prayer

Abba, Father, we're trying to hang on to hope, but it seems we'll never have another child. So much loss and sorrow. Why aren't we allowed to have the family we desire? We're good parents and we have tremendous love to give. Lord, we're begging you to hear our cry and show us your face. Amen.

REVISITING PAIN

Mommy guilt was rising. No one wants an only child! —Laurie

(Except the parents who have none.)

HANNAH WAS IN DEEP ANGUISH, CRYING BITTERLY AS SHE PRAYED TO THE LORD. AND SHE MADE THIS VOW: "O LORD OF HEAVEN'S ARMIES, IF YOU WILL LOOK UPON MY SORROW AND ANSWER MY PRAYER AND GIVE ME A SON, THEN I WILL GIVE HIM BACK TO YOU. HE WILL BE YOURS FOR HIS ENTIRE LIFETIME.
—1 Samuel 1:10–11 NLT

Shannon's Journal

Dear God,

Our family was so excited for us to have another baby, and they're devastated and grieve with us. Each time we try, they become cautiously excited. We're not telling many people until we're further along, but we need help with Joshua and we need prayers.

We hear so often, with a pained expression, "Oh, I hope it works out this time." Or others minimize our pain with, "At least you have Joshua." God, this isn't a consolation. I don't understand why you let others plan and choose how many kids to have, and I don't have that choice. I've started asking people if they would be content with just one, or if they too would feel the pains of wanting another child and feeling their family wasn't yet complete.

God, I'm surprised all my old feelings come up from my struggles to have Josh—the stuff I had set aside when I finally felt "normal" because I was part of the "mommy culture." Trying again and having multiple miscarriages causes me to revisit my previous heartache and pain and now have a bunch of new added sadness. It's a double whammy and feels overwhelming at times.

Each new attempt brings its own set of baggage: past failures and dread mixed with hope and anticipation. In our devastation, we needed to be around couples who understood what we were feeling, so we attended the Grief Support Group at church. God, they gave us a packet of resources and information about grief that described exactly what we were going through!

Each week had a topic for us to discuss. Nobody belittled our loss. They gave us a book about loss and hope and had a balloon-releasing ceremony signifying a step in our letting go and a step toward hope for the future. Thank you for this wonderful group and for dear friends I can walk with through this.

Grieving again, Shannon

A Mommy-in-Waiting Shares

When my husband and I married, we talked about having four more kids: I had a child from a previous marriage. I became pregnant right away, and we have a beautiful ten-year-old daughter. When we revisited thoughts of having another baby, I got pregnant, but at week eight and shortly before Mother's Day, we lost Morgan. I cried violently to the point of wailing.

By September, we were pregnant and hopeful again. But at seven weeks, they were unable to get Michael's heart rate or a good ultrasound. February, I was pregnant yet again. At seven weeks, we had a heart rate, and believing we were safe, started preparing for a baby.

At the ten-week ultrasound, we still had a heart rate and the baby's measurements were good. I took my daughter Ellen with me to my doctor's visit a week later. Everything was going good this time, and I thought this was educational for her. But the doctor gave a long speech ending with, "I think this is another miscarriage." I emerged from the dressing room to find my daughter sobbing. At that moment I realized it was her baby, too. —Laurie

Janet's Mentoring Moment

Laurie did eventually get pregnant again and carried Chloe to full term. Laurie found solace in naming her miscarried babies and wrote a poem for each one. Shannon and Mommy-in-Waiting Sharon also wrote poetry, and Shannon journaled to God. I hope you've been writing your letters to God in the space provided in each chapter. Writing or journaling is a healing way to express feelings as you work through the Stages of Grief, page 267.

God's Love Letter to You

Dear_____ and_____,

I will give you my message in the form of a vision. Write it clearly enough to be read at a glance (Hab. 2:2 CEV).

Your visionary, God

Couple's Prayer

Father, Our sorrow isn't just about us. Other children and extended family are in pain, too. Please comfort them. They grieve with us, and they grieve for a sibling or grandchild that might have been. Lord, in our efforts to complete our family, we remember that we are complete in you. We know you welcomed our lost babies into your loving arms, and we look forward to our family being reunited in our heavenly home with you. Amen.

Your Letter to God

Maybe you'll write a poem or words to a song, but whatever words you write will be music to God's ears. Try releasing to God those children he took directly into his presence. He's waiting to hear your heart and heal your troubled soul.

Dear God, _____ *Date:* _____

_____

_____

_____

_____

_____

_____

_____

_____

_____

_____

_____

_____

_____

_____

_____

_____

Chapter Seventeen

LIVING WITH INFERTILITY

YOU WILL SHOW ME THE WAY OF LIFE,
GRANTING ME THE JOY OF YOUR PRESENCE
AND THE PLEASURES OF LIVING WITH YOU FOREVER.
—Psalm 16:11 NLT

It's a Process

The time it took to become a parent was like the time it would take to pour all the water in the ocean out of a tiny funnel. —Mandy

FRIENDS, WHEN LIFE GETS REALLY DIFFICULT, DON'T JUMP TO THE CONCLUSION THAT GOD ISN'T ON THE JOB. INSTEAD, BE GLAD THAT YOU ARE IN THE VERY THICK OF WHAT CHRIST EXPERIENCED. THIS IS A SPIRITUAL REFINING PROCESS, WITH GLORY JUST AROUND THE CORNER.
—1 Peter 4:12–13 *The Message*

Kim's Journal

Dear God,

After Toby got off work one day, we made the two and a half hour drive to attend Bethany Christian Service's informational meeting where we heard about how the agency connects birth moms with "forever families." Their ministry assists infertile adoptive parents, but primarily they mentor, coach, and care for young pregnant girls and women by helping them make a plan for their unborn babies.

All adoptions through Bethany are open—the birthmother selects an adoptive family from a profile and meets with them at the Bethany office. If everyone wants to proceed with the adoption, they agree on a level of future contact. Some adoptive families remain close with their birthmother, like she's an extended family member, while others stick to a basic agreement of sending pictures and letters with arranged visits at the birthmother's request and adoptive parents' convenience. The adoptive family has access to the baby's family history. This all sounded exciting to us, and we were ready to find out more.

The next step was attending a daylong Adoption Orientation where we learned more details about the adoption process, the adoption tax credit, and the payment schedule. We would need to complete a lengthy application, a home study, background checks, a CPR and first aid course, and a home safety inspection. We joked that we would be more prepared to have a baby than most people.

Finally, after completing those requirements, we'd put together our scrapbook-type profile to show birthmothers. We saw colorful samples marketing prospective parents' likeability with pictures of them doing fun activities and events with extended family. The idea is to make your profile stand out from the others and click with a birthmother. It looked like a fun project.

Then our profile goes into the agency book of profiles, and we begin the waiting game. We were told it could take a week to two years to be chosen by a birthmother, depending on our openness to race and special needs. Wow, this is quite a process, but we're signing up for it! *Going through the process, Kim*

A Mommy-in-Waiting Shares

Our journey to adoption started after several humbling and costly failed attempts with fertility treatments. We had discussed adoption, but we didn't feel the time was right and weren't comfortable with the expense and possible travel to a foreign land. So we prayed for direction. A family friend who had adopted a beautiful little girl from Kazakhstan heard about our plight. Wanting to adopt again, she invited me to attend an adoption seminar with her. I was reluctant, but I went, and it was informative.

One agency continued to resurface: Safe Havens of Kornerstone, a Christian nonprofit foster and adoption agency out of Arlington, Texas. Kornerstone works directly with Child Protective Services to remove at-risk children and place them in safe environments. Donald and I discussed our options, prayed, and eventually decided to call Kornerstone. We felt led to go this route instead of a traditional adoption mainly for monetary reasons, but we also felt a strong connection to the children in our area. We soon knew this would be beyond a life-changing experience; it would be soul-searching and teach us more about each other and what we truly wanted. —Cindy

Janet's Mentoring Moment

The journey from infertility to parenthood involves a process—steps you wouldn't be taking had you become parents naturally. Each step requires prayer and emotional, spiritual, and financial agreement with the process and the progression. If either of you still longs for what could've or should've been, the process will seem like drudgery.

If you can gratefully look at each step as an opportunity, the process could be an adventure leading to the fulfillment of your heart's desire: a child.

God's Love Letter to You

*Dear*_____ *and*_____,

Forgetting what is behind and straining toward what is ahead, press on toward the goal to win the prize for which I, God, have called you heavenward in Christ Jesus. All of you who are mature should take such a view of things. And if on some point you think differently, that too I, God, will make clear to you (Phil. 3:13–15, paraphrased).
On the journey with you, God

Couple's Prayer

Heavenly Father, This journey can be wearying and draining. We want a baby, and there are so many hoops to jump through, procedures, tests, forms to fill out, and decisions to make. But Lord, we know when we hold a child in our arms, this will all be a story in the making. A brief moment compared to the years ahead of loving our child. Give us hope. Help us endure. Amen.

WHERE WERE THOSE YOU EXPECTED TO BE THERE?

I felt alienated from my family. —Michele

THERE IS A FRIEND WHO STICKS CLOSER THAN A BROTHER.
—Proverbs 18:24

Shannon's Journal

Dear God,
After the miscarriages, people say, "I'm deeply sorry for your loss." But I want them to visit, spend time, and compassionately ask, "How are you?" Lord, some people do "get it" and are supportive, and I can share my personal and private stories.

I asked you to bring a friend to talk to. Someone who would understand and validate how I felt and let me be honest. Thank you for the gift of the special friend I met in the Grief Support Group. We went on weekly walks, pouring out our hearts and pain to each other. We shared our anger with you, God, and our hope to be in a better place one day. We talked about the black cloud hanging over us, and how we wished to be anywhere but here at this point in our lives.

We talked about our walk with you. I know you heard the prayers we prayed for each other and our endless talks on the phone.
Grateful for my special friend, Shannon

A Mommy-in-Waiting Shares

Words can't describe seeing the beautiful heartbeat of our baby at seven weeks. All pain was forgotten. Added to the excitement, my best friend Julie told me she was pregnant that same week with her first baby after trying to conceive for over a year. Five days after seeing our baby's heartbeat, I began to spot and lost the baby.

When once words couldn't describe our joy, now words couldn't describe our sorrow. I was a wreck. It was too difficult being around Julie and her husband, whose pregnancy was going on without incident. Every time I saw her growing stomach, I'd think of how big my stomach should be. They were experiencing the most exciting and happy time of their lives, while we were terribly sad. I believed nobody knew my pain . . . not even God.

In my despair, I called a family member for consolation. In an attempt to "fix" my emotions, I heard, "It was *only* a miscarriage." "Worse things can happen." "Perhaps your stress caused the miscarriage." And "If you lose your friendship with Julie, it's your own fault." If my own family couldn't comprehend my grief, how could the God of the Universe?

When I found out Julie was having a girl, I cried for an hour and then confessed my jealousy to the Lord. But when my niece informed my sister she was pregnant by a boy she knew, I cried for a week. It was a tremendous hardship to my sister, but I couldn't be a support to her. All I comprehended was that my niece would be bringing the next baby into the family, and I wouldn't. —Michele

Janet's Mentoring Moment

Often people you expect to provide comfort in a crisis don't, and ones you least expect do. Shannon said she learned a valuable truth: people usually aren't trying to be insensitive. They simply don't understand something they haven't experienced. Rather than feeling hurt or misunderstood, pray for "clueless" people to develop compassion surpassing their own comprehension, because they're missing the blessing of being a blessing. Pray you'll do the same when you're the clueless person or aren't available for someone who needs your support.

While the disappointment is real with those who let you down, thanking God for the ones who come through for you replaces sadness with gladness.

God's Love Letter to You

*Dear*_____ *and*_____,
Be merciful just as I, your Father, am merciful. Do not judge, and you will not be judged. Do not condemn, and you will not be condemned. Forgive, and you will be forgiven (Luke 6:36–37, paraphrased).
Your forgiver, God

Couple's Prayer

Merciful Savior, Thank you for forgiving us the many times we've let you down. You never condemn us or make us feel guilty. Lord, help us be merciful to those who disappoint us, and keep our minds centered on those who pleasantly surprise us. You are a merciful and forgiving God, filled with grace and love. Let us go and do likewise. In your gracious name we pray. Amen.

SO MANY DISAPPOINTMENTS

We prepared ourselves to be disappointed again. We were getting
very good at being disappointed! The birthmother chose to keep the
baby, and we didn't lose anything except some hope and gained some
experience for the next time. —Sharon

What kept me going through the disappointments was my faith that
all things work together for the good of those who love God and
are called according to his purpose. So I know his plan is best
even though it hurts a lot. —Mandy

AND WE KNOW THAT IN ALL THINGS GOD WORKS FOR THE GOOD OF THOSE
WHO LOVE HIM, WHO HAVE BEEN CALLED ACCORDING TO HIS PURPOSE.
—Romans 8:28

Shannon's Journal

Dear God,
I feel like I'm always writing sad thoughts about disappointments. Today we had a doctor's appointment to use our last round of frozen embryos for our *third* try. Could I have prepared more? I heard the hurt and bitterness in our voices. God, help the staff to understand and be

patient. Do we need to have hope and enthusiasm to do this again, or is a glimmer of expectation enough?

I was surprised by the emotions that came up—such sadness pulling into the fertility clinic parking lot. I felt discouraged and defeated. The nurses and doctor said so many positive and encouraging things, yet I felt no excitement. Is this what people mean when they say you don't invest in the pregnancy until you get past the point where you lost the last one?

I'm scared I'll never feel a baby in my womb or see my belly grow big again. I don't understand what's happening. I can't see what you see. Why does it feel like it's never my turn? It seems so unfair. Years of hurt and disappointment, for what? At least help me see.

God, I know you know my heart's desires, so I'm writing it all down, putting it in your hands. If you're not going to give us a baby again through IVF, then give me new desires. Heal my heart. Come, do your work. Help me let go and move on. May adoption sound sweeter and sweeter to my soul.

Discouraged, Shannon

A Mommy-in-Waiting Shares

I came to my own conclusion that since we didn't get pregnant with all the fertility treatments, we probably weren't able to have children, although the doctor couldn't confirm this. My emotional pain and disappointment from not conceiving led to hidden envy when other women—especially those I deemed unfit for children—got pregnant. I couldn't attend baby showers or watch commercials with babies. I even ended a friendship because I was angry and jealous that she got pregnant under unfavorable circumstances. I became judgmental and hard-hearted.

In my pursuit to fulfill something I wanted, I inadvertently made an idol out of my desire for a baby. When the Lord exposed my heart, I repented and literally opened my hands and vowed to love and serve him all my life, even if he never allowed me to have a baby. About a year and a half later, I was pregnant and gave birth to a beautiful baby boy. —Tressia

Janet's Mentoring Moment

Disappointing treatments, procedures, or adoption attempts make it difficult to believe anything good *ever* will happen. Admittedly, discouragements accompany the infertility journey, but encouragements tag along, too. Don't let the negative overshadow the positive. There's no fear, obstacle, pain, doubt, worry, or disappointment too big for God to overcome. Expect it. Believe it. Pray for it. God will never disappoint you: that's encouraging!

God's Love Letter to You

Dear_____ and_____,

Unrelenting disappointment leaves you heartsick, but a sudden good break can turn life around (Prov. 13:12 *The Message*).

Provider of good breaks, God

Couple's Prayer

Father, You know better than anyone the disappointments and letdowns we've experienced. Help us hold on to you when our world is crashing. Help us keep a positive perspective that things could take a turn for the better when we wake up tomorrow. And if they don't, we'll keep our eyes on the next tomorrow. Amen.

YOU NEED AN OUTLET

Our new business was the perfect gift. This was our "baby" before God gave us our real baby to raise and love. Wow—it reminds me not to push or rush God in his planning. —Karen

OBSESSION WITH SELF IN THESE MATTERS IS A DEAD END; ATTENTION TO GOD LEADS US OUT INTO THE OPEN, INTO A SPACIOUS, FREE LIFE. FOCUSING ON THE SELF IS THE OPPOSITE OF FOCUSING ON GOD. ANYONE COMPLETELY ABSORBED IN SELF IGNORES GOD, ENDS UP THINKING MORE ABOUT SELF THAN GOD. THAT PERSON IGNORES WHO GOD IS AND WHAT HE IS DOING. AND GOD ISN'T PLEASED AT BEING IGNORED.
—Romans 8:6–8 *The Message*

Shannon's Journal

Dear God,

Well, the third IVF ended in another miscarriage. We need to take a break from trying to have another baby and being disappointed. I prayed if you're shutting this door in my life for now, please show me what you want me to do with my time.

I heard you say to start back to school, so I finished my bachelor's degree and discovered my career path and love for speech therapy. Working as a speech therapist helped remind me there is more to my life and me than this experience of infertility. Infertility is part of my life, a bump in the road, but it doesn't define me or my identity.

More than infertile, Shannon

A Mommy-in-Waiting Shares

We knew we needed to adopt or do embryo adoption after Ken's Sertoli-cell-only syndrome (SCO) diagnosis—a one in a million condition. Almost like we were handpicked by God. OK, so *our* plan obviously wasn't what God had intended for us. And then it happened: I was moving forward in life. I felt like the path God had me on was no longer narrow and winding; it was six feet wide and straight. So I quit my job I wasn't enjoying, took six months to write a business plan, secured funding, and launched my own business. Today Ken and I both work at our business while raising our daughter. —Karen

Janet's Mentoring Moment

Shannon came to an important realization: there was more to life than trying to have a baby, which can become all-consuming if you let it. Say with Shannon: "Infertility doesn't define me. It's not my identity."

What were your interests before infertility took over your life? What are you good at? What do you enjoy doing as a couple? Do all those things now. There's a good chance you've lost interest in many things that gave your life meaning and dimension. Or maybe it's time to try a new venture that requires thinking and focusing on something besides infertility treatments or filling out adoption papers.

God's Love Letter to You

Dear_____ and_____ ,

You should use whatever gift you have received from me to serve others, faithfully administering my grace in its various forms. If you speak, do it as one speaking my very words. If you serve, do it with the strength I, God, provide, so that in all things I may be praised through my Son, Jesus Christ. To him be the glory and the power for ever and ever (1 Pet. 4:10–11, paraphrased).

Creative gift giver, God

Couple's Prayer

Lord God, We admit our lives have become one-dimensional. Everything we do centers on having a baby. Help us reconnect with each other and the things that bring us joy, pleasure, and fulfillment. Lord, we know you gifted us with talents other than being parents. Please let us rediscover those interests and maybe develop new ones. Remind us of the people we were before setting out on this journey. Help us find our way back to you and to each other. Amen.

MAINTAINING HOPE

I want and need a glimmer of hope. —Shannon

WHY ARE YOU DOWNCAST, O MY SOUL? WHY SO DISTURBED WITHIN
ME? PUT YOUR HOPE IN GOD, FOR I WILL YET PRAISE HIM, MY
SAVIOR AND MY GOD.
—Psalm 42:5–6

Kim's Journal

Dear God,

At the Bethany orientation meeting, we listened to a panel of birthmothers share their stories. They had been pregnant teenagers not ready to raise a child. All had different levels of contact with the adoptive families and none regretted their decision. The Christian-based counseling at Bethany prepared them to put their babies up for adoption. Our view of a woman who would make such a decision changed after hearing their stories. These women loved their children and wanted the best for them.

We also heard from a panel of adoptive families and their forever children. This was exciting because we saw the end result, and the children were adorable. We heard about the couples' infertility struggles while desperately wanting a child and the exciting moment they received "the call" they were going to be parents. Some were even in the labor room when their babies were born. We really wanted a newborn, and the thought of possibly being present when our baby took his or her first breath was more than we imagined.

We left that day with a new sense of hope. We *really* were going to be parents. It wasn't happening the way we imagined, but you hadn't given up on us. We knew you would be at work connecting us with our child.

Hopefully, Kim

A Mommy-in-Waiting Shares

We wrote our "birthmother letter" describing ourselves, outlining our hobbies (specifically, four-wheeling), and praying the letter would bless whoever read it and give them peace in their decisions. With the help of friends and family, we passed out our profile to contacts familiar with the adoption process. The next two years were full of wondering, praying, growing, disappointment, anger, confusion, doubt. . . . The emptiness grew deeper and darker each day.

Then we began feeling hopeful and trusting God was working on something wonderful. We received a call that a birthmother due in February had chosen us, but to our disappointment it didn't work out. February stuck in our minds as we struggled with taking other avenues, but my husband had faith God was going to use us, and it wasn't for us to control.

Finally, we received another call from the Pregnancy Crisis Center. We had been "chosen" by a birthmother in prison who was being released in January and due for a cesarean section February fifth! She loved our profile, especially the common interest in four-wheeling. When we met her, we felt God's presence as we connected and excitedly talked like family of *our* baby's future birth. What we weren't expecting was Satan's plan to create obstacles to test our faith, but nothing could deter us. During one of my breakdowns, a good friend reminded me that God doesn't start anything he doesn't finish. It was what God knew I needed to hear. —Jackie

Janet's Mentoring Moment

God is your only reliable source of hope—not doctors, researchers, scientists, counselors, family, agencies, spouses—they're simply the instruments God uses for fulfilling desires. Stay prayerful and hopeful, and believe that God will change your situation. "Happy are those who have the God of Israel as their helper, whose hope is in the Lord their God. He is the one who made heaven and earth, the sea, and everything in them. He is the one who keeps every promise forever" (Ps. 146:5–6 NLT).

Here are ways to maintain life-sustaining hope when things *seem* hopeless:

- Don't keep company with unsupportive people.
- Ask your family and friends to join you in hopeful, positive, productive discussion.
- Think expectantly about the possible before dismissing something as impossible.
- Ask everyone you know to pray *expectantly* and *hopefully*.
- Consider redefining your goal.

God's Love Letter to You

Dear_____and_____,

Always continue to fear me, the Lord. For surely you have a future ahead of you; your hope will not be disappointed. My children, listen and be wise. Keep your hearts on the right course (Prov. 23:17–19 NLT, paraphrased).

Your wellspring of hope, God

Couple's Prayer

Precious Lord, Since we have been justified through faith, we have peace with God through our Lord Jesus Christ, through whom we have gained access by faith into this grace in which we now stand. And we rejoice in the hope of the glory of God. Not only so, but we also rejoice in our sufferings, because we know that suffering produces perseverance; perseverance, character; and character, hope. And hope does not disappoint us, because God has poured out his love into our hearts by the Holy Spirit, whom he has given us. Amen. (Rom. 5:1–5)

MANAGING STRESS AND RELEASING PARALYZING FEAR

The fear of the unknown and the doubting was the Devil's favorite weapon. Fear was preventing us from loving the child God had chosen for us. —Cindy

CAN ALL YOUR WORRIES ADD A SINGLE MOMENT TO YOUR LIFE? AND IF WORRY CAN'T ACCOMPLISH A LITTLE THING LIKE THAT, WHAT'S THE USE OF WORRYING OVER BIGGER THINGS?
—Luke 12:25–26 NLT

Kim's Journal

Dear God,

Checking off things on our adoption "to do" list was therapeutic. Until now, everything seemed out of our control, but finally, it felt like we had some control over our situation. The quicker we got through the checklists, courses, and paperwork, the quicker we become parents. I had us moving along.

Selecting pictures for our profile was enjoyable, even with numerous trips to Kinko's to make copies. I found creative scissors for scalloping picture edges and bought construction paper for framing. I chose bright yellow stationery bordered with gerbera daisies and stickers to decorate the pages. I wanted our profile to stand out from the rest—eye-catching and fun, yet tasteful—a representation of a loving family for a child.

We needed five identical profiles for each Bethany office in our state and fifteen extra biography pages for birthmothers to take home. Each profile was seven pages, front and back, plus the biography page. A lot of pictures, paper, stickers, cutting, gluing, and . . . time. I started this project full of excitement, anticipation, and energy, but as the weeks went on, I felt stressed and out of control again. I feared never completing the profiles. The longer it took, the longer for me to become a mother. The pressure became overwhelming. This was the only thing standing between me and my future baby. I was irritable and short-tempered with everyone close to me.

Thanksgiving was coming up, and we were hosting both sides of our family for the long weekend. I'd have to put away this project that had overtaken my life. While I was looking forward to everyone's visit, it seemed like one more setback in my lengthy journey.

My mom sensed my preoccupation. When I confessed the pressure I felt and the time it was taking to complete the profiles, she and my mother-in-law offered to help. I was excited. This could actually be fun again. I got out my supplies, and we began an assembly line of cutting, pasting, and sticking. For two days, we sat around the table talking, laughing, and enjoying each other's company. When everyone left, my project was complete. Thank you, Lord, for my supportive family.

Monday morning as I mailed the profiles to Bethany, a huge weight lifted from my shoulders. Our part was done; now we wait and pray.

Feeling lighter, Kim

A Mommy-in-Waiting Shares

When the foster and adoption agency came to interview us the first time, we cleaned house for days. What we've come to realize is that a lot of people come to your home before an adoption can take place. In the interview when they asked, "How did you become Christians?" I smiled, thinking: *This feels very right.*

We anxiously started the classes required for becoming foster or adoptive parents, but after completion, we did nothing! It was March, then August, then November, and still we did nothing. I don't know what we were waiting on—a baby to knock on our door, perhaps. I think we were afraid of the unknown. We wanted so badly to be in the center of God's will, and we didn't want to mess things up. Were we reading God's signals right? Maybe we were being selfish? My girlfriends encouraged, "Just do it! If it's not right, God won't let it happen."

Finally, we decided to "Just do it." We were off with background checks, cabinet locks, CPR classes, outlet covers, proof of insurance, locking up meds, pet vaccinations, gun safes, fire escape plans, and health inspections. The family developer came to the house for the grueling six-hour home study where we told our life stories. They know our blood types and whether we're a boxer or briefs family. Finally, we were licensed one month short of a year from completing the original classes. We didn't break any speed record, that's for sure! —Cindy

Janet's Mentoring Moment

Satan's favorite tactics—overwhelming tasks, stress, anxiety, and fear—paralyzed Kim and Cindy. Satan uses these effective ploys to foil our realization of God's wonderful plans for us. We sabotage our own dream. What Satan doesn't count on is God sending in reinforcements. Both Kim and Cindy shared their stress and concerns with others and accepted help and encouragement to keep moving toward their heart's desire: a child.

God's Love Letter to You

Dear_____ and_____,

Humble yourselves under my mighty power, and in my good time, I will honor you. Give all your worries and cares to me, God, for I care about what happens to you. Be careful! Watch out for attacks from the devil, your great enemy. He prowls around like a roaring lion, looking for some victim to devour. Take a firm stand against him, and be strong in your faith (1 Pet. 5:6–9 NLT, paraphrased).

Your stress-buster, God

Couple's Prayer

Lord, Slowly we're learning about our "new normal" life of infertility and what we need to do to navigate through unknown territory. Often we feel overwhelmed, stressed, fearful . . . and wonder if it's worth all the work and headaches. But, Lord, you put this dream and desire in our hearts to be parents, and with your help, we're staying the course. Amen.

BEING A GOOD WITNESS

Pray with and for us that our faith would be unwavering, we would know and see God's goodness through everything, and we as a family would be a testimony of God's faithfulness and love. —Tiffany and Simon

I WILL PRAISE THE LORD AT ALL TIMES. I WILL CONSTANTLY
SPEAK HIS PRAISES. I WILL BOAST ONLY IN THE LORD; LET ALL
WHO ARE DISCOURAGED TAKE HEART. COME, LET US TELL OF
THE LORD'S GREATNESS; LET US EXALT HIS NAME TOGETHER.
—Psalm 34:1–3 NLT

Shannon's Journal

Dear God,
I believe being a good witness is being honest about where I'm at and taking everything to you—the good, the bad, the ugly . . . my trust, my mistrust, my doubts, my fears—all of it. Sure, I get bitter and resentful and cry out, "It isn't fair," but that's usually when my hurt is rising to the surface, and I need a good cry. You truly have met me in many pits in my life, and that's what I want to remember and share with others.
Honestly, Shannon

A Mommy- and Daddy-in-Waiting Share

In the midst of our deepest grief at the loss of baby Ezekiel, we don't regret our embryo adoption experience. Yes, it was unfair and too short; yet, how can we complain about twenty-five weeks of having Ezekiel grow inside Tiff? How could we regret the experience of loving him by preparing his nursery and the blessing of God's people praying for him? Was the diagnosis of hydrocephalus for us to love him more? The experience of loving Ezekiel is irreplaceable. He is our son.

We know for certain God remains in control and is sovereign. His plans are better than ours, even when they don't make sense and life is hard. Through many emotional and spiritual ups and downs, we've learned so much about God's character and our own. God puts surprises in our lives, but never more than we can handle.

While our hearts praise him, our minds question: "How much more, Lord? Haven't we learned what you wanted us to learn? Aren't we glorifying you through our lives as living testimonies of your loving-kindness and strength?"

How God brings us through this will bring glory to him. We can't imagine going through something like this without faith, because the hope we have wouldn't exist. By faith, we know God is still good and worthy of our deepest

praise. As for his name, Ezekiel, we still require God's strength for comfort.
—Tiffany and Simon (Excerpt from a Christmas letter and eulogy for Ezekiel)

Janet's Mentoring Moment

Tiffany and Simon chose to use their tragic loss as a witness and testimony to friends and family. They admit to questioning God, while still praising him and helping others view their circumstances through God's eyes. Christ in your heart allows you to see God glorified through the hurt and pain. What a witness to others watching to see how Christians go through trials—do we fall apart like the world often does by turning to alcohol, drugs, cheating, or leaving? Or do we admit pain and sorrow but still proclaim trust and confidence in our sovereign God?

Sometimes Christians mistakenly think they always have to smile and maintain a Pollyanna attitude. It's OK to feel sad and mad. God knows how you feel, and he'll comfort you. That's what others will see: Christians experience bad things like everyone else, but they handle their pain with grace and hope. Others will ask how you endure this hardship, and the door is open to share the hope and peace of Christ living in your heart, which is available to them, too.

God's Love Letter to You

Dear_____ and_____,
If someone asks about your Christian hope, always be ready to explain it. But do this in a gentle and respectful way (1 Pet. 3:15-16a NLT).
Your Hope, God

Couple's Prayer

Oh Lord, Please let us remain hopeful and be a good witness to family, friends, doctors . . . whomever you put in our path. We can't do this without you giving us the strength and determination to sing your praises when our hearts are breaking. Show us your ways, Lord. Give us your strength. We put our lives and our future family into your capable hands. Amen.

Your Letter to God

How are you dealing with the process and disappointments? Who could help or pray for you to keep moving in the right direction to becoming parents? How can your infertility journey be a witness to God's goodness? How are you maintaining hope?

Dear God,   *Date:*
_____

_____

_____

_____

_____

_____

_____

_____

_____

_____

_____

_____

_____

_____

_____

_____

_____

_____

_____

_____

_____

Chapter Eighteen

RELYING ON GOD

So we're not giving up. How could we!
Even though on the outside it often looks
like things are falling apart on us,
on the inside, where God is making new life,
not a day goes by without his unfolding grace.
These hard times are small potatoes compared to the coming good times,
the lavish celebration prepared for us.
There's far more here than meets the eye.
The things we see now are here today, gone tomorrow.
But the things we can't see now will last forever.
—2 Corinthians 4:16–18 *The Message*

Infertility Tests Your Faith

Know that God holds you, regardless of how you feel about him right now. Even when you feel your faith has failed, he's praying for you that you will not be sifted down to nothing.—Anissa, comforting her sister and brother-in-law at their stillborn's funeral

Our faith has definitely been tested and strengthened. —Simon and Tiffany

I couldn't tell you when we stopped talking to God. It was so gradual. We even stopped talking to each other about it. I stopped reading my Bible and doing devotions. —Mel

Now faith is being sure of what we hope for and certain of what we do not see.
—Hebrews 11:1

Shannon's Journal

Dear God,
I want to start praying again for my next child. At this point, I welcome more than one. You know my heart, God. You know I ache to be pregnant again, to have a sibling for Joshua.

Sometimes I think about my many shortcomings and faults and wonder if that's why I don't have another child. I know you can take care of those thoughts, so I must write them down to get them out of my mind.

First, I feel like we can barely afford the child we have, and I have bad days when I run out of patience and energy. I can be very selfish sometimes. I know others have bad days, too, but I get down on myself. Then, it's hard when my friends have had more children and completed their families. I feel passed by. I can't relate to them as I used to.

So I question myself and my relationships. I equate these things to my value as a mom, and for some reason I hold on to these thoughts more than I look to you. I must tell you all this so it doesn't fester inside me, because they are untruths, not nearly fitting for how you see me and my gifts. Remove them from my mind, God. I'm scared to try again. Calm me. Reassure me. I don't think I've ever been more surrendered into your hands until now. My life, my future is truly yours. I have no money left or credit to make decisions with . . . only you can make another child happen.

Thank you for the special people who see things I don't, like my sister-in-law's continual encouragement that she sees me having more kids. She has faith for me during my dark days. It's like that song by Bebo Norman, "If your faith is hard to find, you can borrow mine."
Faithfully yours, Shannon

A Mommy-in-Waiting Shares

I felt incapable—my self-esteem crushed by not being able to do what a woman's body was made to do. My heart was sick, and I started to feel weak and useless. This was my continual thought pattern for several months as I prayed and cried and prayed some more. I trusted God to supply my needs and to be faithful to his promises, but I didn't see or understand how or why infertility fit into his plan. His Word says he wants to give us the desires of our hearts. Yet I knew that in his sovereignty, he knew what was best for me, and I feared it might not include children. What hurt more than anything was knowing that God knew I was hurting, and it seemed he didn't care. He was silent. —Danette

A Daddy-in-Waiting Shares

We lost our first baby through an ectopic pregnancy. Less than a year later, our identical twins died at eight weeks' gestation. Again, our hopes dashed—this time twice over! As Christians, God's predestined people, it might be natural to ask how our Creator, with whom we are in a right relationship through Christ, could allow such devastating trials into our lives.

My wife Amy and I wondered, *God, if we're serving you, then how can you allow these children to die?* How often do we, his creatures, demand answers from our Creator? Besides, how can God's glory possibly be revealed in our suffering? The answers are in his Word. While we might question why and when God orchestrates life circumstances, we are to commit ourselves to our "faithful Creator and continue to do good" (1 Pet. 4:19). That's what we *chose* to do! Even though we had Job-like questions, we continued to do good while clinging to 2 Corinthians 12:9, "My grace is sufficient for you, for my power is made perfect in weakness."
—Adam McManus

Janet's Mentoring Moment

You may be asking: If God loves me, why isn't he doing something? Then you feel guilty for waning faith in God and his timing. It's a downward spiral fueled by living in an impatient "now" society, where it's not easy waiting on God's response to your situation. Your deadline passes—maybe it's another birthday or the timeline you set for having a baby—and you think God has forgotten about you or you haven't prayed enough or prayed for the right things. You consider intervening to change your situation.

Faith believes in God when he can't be seen or heard. Sometimes God tests our faith by making us wait longer than we would like, or he goes silent for awhile, but he never stops believing in us. God honors faithfulness. When plans seem unclear, wisdom waits. Act on God's certain promises, not chancy probabilities. Remember: God is the solution, not the problem!

God's Love Letter to You

*Dear*_____*and*_____,
Stay on your toes. Satan has tried his best to separate all of you from me, like chaff from wheat. I've prayed for you in particular that you not give in or give out (Luke 22:31-32 *The Message,* paraphrased).
Faithfully yours, God

Couple's Prayer

Please Lord, Help us maintain our faith and believe that you *are* working in our best interests. We don't understand, and yet you tell us that faith is just that—believing in things we cannot comprehend and see. God, there are times when our faith wavers—in you, ourselves, our ability to parent. We doubt you and we doubt ourselves. We know this isn't a good place for our thoughts to camp, but when our hopes are dashed, we wonder why you're letting this happen. Keep us faithful, Lord, to you and to each other. Amen.

TRUSTING GOD

Some days it was all I could do to get out of bed and put one foot in front of the other. I had to decide every day whether I trusted the goodness of the God of the universe. —Sarah

Trust God's purpose in your life. He will amaze you! —Danette

DO NOT LET YOUR HEARTS BE TROUBLED. TRUST IN GOD; TRUST ALSO IN ME [JESUS].
—John 14:1

Shannon's Journal

Dear God,

Taking breaks between treatments gave me a chance to gather myself back together and renew my hope after so many disappointments. Getting involved in ministry and women's small groups really helped because I could see you answering the women's prayers and doing good things in their lives, and it reminded me of the times you did that for me. It helped me draw near to you and trust in what you were doing and what you wanted to tell me. I felt encouraged that good times were ahead for me also. These people prayed for me, and I felt their prayers.

I also started to see how you were doing things and moving in my life; not in the way I wanted, but still working, still there, still holding on to me when I backed away or lost a bit of my trust. Ministry changed my focus as I thought about something else besides having another baby, if just for an hour. It reminded me of other gifts you've given me.

I've always had a deep belief that you told me in vitro could work, and I can't let go of the dream, even as we pursue adoption.

Believing, Shannon

A Mommy-in-Waiting Shares

God showed me repeatedly that he was only asking me to be faithful. My heart felt him saying: *Danette, you don't have to know or understand what I am doing, just trust me! My ways are not your ways, and my thoughts are not your thoughts. For you* *know that in all things I work for the good of those who love me, who have been called* *according to my purpose. My purpose, Danette, not yours! Let go of this dream; lay it* *at my feet and be willing to walk away. Like Abraham and Isaac, you have to trust me* *completely*. I knew that my God was good, no matter what. I knew he heard my cry, and whether or not he answered my prayers for children, I could and would still faithfully trust him. —Danette

Janet's Mentoring Moment

Why would God ask Danette to let go of her dream? Bruce Wilkinson has the answer, "The time will come when God asks you to surrender the Dream itself. If you don't surrender your Dream, you will be placing it higher on your priority list than God. You will go forward from this moment with a break in your relationship with your Dream Giver. Your Dream will become your idol. But your Dream—no matter how big—will make a tiny god."[1]

Trusting God is easy when everything is going great, and he's readily answering our heart's desires. The real challenge comes when we have no idea what God is doing. It's hard to trust God's plan when we want what we want when we want it, and he doesn't seem to be coming through. Like Danette, trust him with your dream anyway. God sees the bigger picture. While not everything that happens *is* good, God can use everything that happens *for* good.

Retrospectively, the couples in this book can see the hand of God in their circumstances and more clearly understand why they went through their trials. They would agree with Tressia, who said, "Of this I am confident: God is worthy of all my love and service because he is God, and my worship is never dependant upon me getting what I want—even if what I want is a good thing. From what we have experienced, I have learned to trust and believe that God is good. When I was able to let go of my bitterness and embrace this mindset, it freed me from the prison of infertility pain."

God's Love Letter to You

Dear_____ and_____,
Trust in me, the Lord, and do good. Then you will live safely in the land and prosper. Take delight in me, the Lord, and I will give you your heart's desires. Commit everything you do to me, the Lord. Trust in me, and I will help you (Ps. 37:3–5 NLT, paraphrased).
I AM trustworthy, God

Couple's Prayer

Our Lord and Dream Giver, We place our complete faith and trust in your Dream and surrender our dream to you. Together we say—"When we get really afraid we come to you in trust. We're proud to praise God; fearless now, we trust in God." Amen (Ps. 56:3–4 *The Message,* paraphrased).

CAN YOU HEAR HIM NOW?

After multiple tests, we had no conclusions, no answers. I needed time to heal emotionally and spiritually. I had so many questions for God. —Michele

I LISTEN CAREFULLY TO WHAT GOD THE LORD IS SAYING,
FOR HE SPEAKS PEACE TO HIS FAITHFUL PEOPLE.
—Psalm 85:8 NLT

Shannon's Journal

Dear God,
When events are too overwhelming, music touches me. Many nights I sit in the dark and listen or sing along to music and cry or journal—especially when I don't know what else to do and feel sad. If the words of a song speak to how I feel, I listen over and over again. This is my time with you, when I tune out all distractions and just sit at your feet, pouring out my heart. Talking to you, I recognize your timing; listening to you, I feel at one with you.

I hear your encouragements throughout the day. My journal has become a promise book where I write meaningful songs, Bible verses, dreams, and feelings to remind me you're there, the future will be good, and you have wonderful plans for me. Interesting how when things are good, I don't draw as near, but during tough times I cling to you.
Listening, Shannon

A Mommy- and Daddy-in-Waiting Share

When Eric and I first learned we couldn't have a biological child, my friend Donna told me about a program called Snowflakes through which you can adopt frozen embryos. I was so distraught I didn't want to hear about anything else, so she dropped the idea.

Months went by and another friend, Lisa, asked me how I was feeling, and I wasn't doing well spiritually or emotionally. She said she had an article she wanted me to read. Three days later, another friend, Janice, approached me with a Focus on the Family article about Snowflakes. Lisa joined us and said that it was the same article!

My husband and I *really* started feeling the power of God! Was this what God wanted for us? I was nervous about the emotions the article would invoke, so I prayed first. As I started reading, I fell to me knees laughing and crying out to God, "This is what you want us to do! You want us to save a life!" It was like God spoke back to me in a very clear voice, "YES, this is what I want you to do!" After sharing this experience with my husband, we prayed like we never prayed before and stepped out in faith to start on our wonderful, emotional journey of embryo adoption. —Eric and Kristina

Janet's Mentoring Moment

God speaks through: music, praying, Scriptures, people, sermons, journaling, articles, circumstances, dreams . . . the list is endless. You feel the leading of the Holy Spirit and sense his presence. Don't always expect a burning bush. God often reveals himself in ordinary experiences. Stay vigilant and don't let "aha!" moments pass as coincidences.

Chris Tiegreen reminds us that when you're seeking God's will, he's revealing it to you: "Do not let the currents of your circumstances dictate the direction you'll take. That's God's domain. His voice is to speak more loudly to us than the boundaries that box us in."[2] You'll hear God clearly when you listen for that still, small voice.

God's Love Letter to You

Dear_____ and_____,
Listen for my voice in everything you do, everywhere you go; I'm the one who will keep you on track. Don't assume that you know it all. Run to me, God (Prov. 3:6–7 *The Message,* paraphrased)!
I AM speaking, God

Couple's Prayer

Praises to you, Lord. We're in awe that you listen to our pleas and speak into our hearts, but we confess we're often not listening. Is it you that wakes us in the middle of the night wanting to talk? Is that the only way you can get our attention? Lord, we want to be more receptive. Intrusive noise often drowns out your gentle whisper. We must make time to be alone with you and still our minds and thoughts. Please provide us moments when all we hear is you. Give us ears to hear and a heart that listens and obeys. Please speak in ways we understand. Remind us to share with others what your voice sounds like so they can hear you, too. Amen.

DRAWING CLOSE TO GOD

I was young in my faith when we first started this process, but our failed first attempt at IVF drew me closer to the Lord. —Paula

BUT AS FOR ME, HOW GOOD IT IS TO BE NEAR GOD! I HAVE MADE THE
SOVEREIGN LORD MY SHELTER, AND I WILL TELL EVERYONE
ABOUT THE WONDERFUL THINGS YOU DO.
—Psalm 73:28 NLT

Kim's Journal

Dear God,

One day when I was crying out to you, something amazing happened. I felt you closer than ever before. I realized I'd never really had a deep conversation with you. It took this infertility heartache to empty me of my own understanding so you could fill me with yours. Our relationship went from surface to intimate and deep as I poured out my heart to you. When I finally put all my trust in you, I felt your comforting embrace. There still are times when I feel sad and alone, but then I hear you tell me you are with me, and I remember this verse: "Trust in the LORD with all your heart and lean not on your own understanding; in all your ways acknowledge him, and he will direct your paths" (Prov. 3:5–6).

We needed you near to direct us in establishing parameters for an adopted baby. It's like placing a special order for a car: we had to decide not just what race we're open to, but the percentages and combinations of different races and the same for special needs and family health. They said to be specific, but limiting our parameters too much would result in a longer wait. Our profile would only be shown to a birthmother matching our criteria. We really had to pray hard about what we were open to in a child. Special needs? Did race matter?

After much prayer and time with you, we feel peace with our choices and confident you will bring a child perfectly matched for our family. As I've come to realize that I want a lifetime of family more than nine months of pregnancy, I see how you've transformed me. I have faith that as you lead us on this adoption journey, you'll be by my side the whole way.

Close to you, Kim

A Mommy- and Daddy-in-Waiting Share

God made it clear that Snowflakes embryo adoption was the journey he had for us. The first attempt didn't result in a pregnancy. We grieved the loss of those four implanted embryos, but the Spirit seemed so close and kept assuring us we were on the right road and to keep going: this was God's plan for us. As I was grieving, I eventually felt a peace that God was using me to be his vessel to send these children home to him. I didn't understand why he didn't let them stay with us, but we kept the faith and continued on our journey trusting we were doing the Lord's will.

We went through a second matching and embryo transfer. After many emotional, spiritual, and physical struggles, we finally have a gift from God we thought was only a dream. We praise him because we wouldn't have it any other way. We love and adore our beautiful daughter, Elise. "Praise God from whom all blessings flow!" —Eric and Kristina

A Mommy-in-Waiting Shares

In the beginning of our infertility journey, my walk with God was somewhat distant—even if he didn't cause the infertility, he certainly didn't stop it. Didn't he love me enough not to want me to hurt so? But I learned that God can be trusted, and he has the best in store for me. 2 Corinthians 4:16–18 was so instrumental in my turnaround, I memorized it. Everything I experience passes through the loving hand of a heavenly Father who wants me to be mindful that this world isn't the end, and everything I go through is to prepare me for eternity. I found myself drawing closer to God and relying on his strength. —Sarah

Janet's Mentoring Moment

It's natural to wonder: Where is God in all this? The answer: He's going through everything with you, and if you let him, he'll show you exciting evidence of his presence. If you're finding it difficult to experience God during your infertility, seek out a couple strong in their faith who have endured a similar experience. Ask them to pray with you and share ways they relied on God in their crisis. Don't be afraid to ask. If they're the right couple, they'll be delighted to spend time encouraging you in the Lord.

God wants us sharing how he was there for us, and he'll be there for others too, just as the couples in this book are sharing with you their crisis of faith and their faith in the crisis. As you begin drawing closer to God—and you will—and grow stronger spiritually—and you will—God will put someone in your life for you to help—and you will.

God's Love Letter to You

Dear_____ and_____,

Draw near to me with a sincere heart in full assurance of faith, having your hearts sprinkled to cleanse you from a guilty conscience and having your bodies washed with pure water. Hold unswervingly to the hope you profess, for I who promised am faithful (Heb. 10:22–23, paraphrased).

Closely, God

Couple's Prayer

Abba, Father, Sometimes one of us doesn't feel close to you. Help us not be resentful or prideful when one feels more spiritual than the other. Let us draw from each other's strengths and extend extra love and prayers to the one who is feeling down. Help us draw closer to you, and to each other, in the good and difficult times. Amen.

WHEN GOD REWRITES YOUR SCRIPT OR ALL IN GOD'S TIMING

Scripture repeatedly reminded me God loved me. Every story of a barren woman I found in Scripture was a miraculous blessing to me. They all were in his control and plan. It was the Lord who opened and closed the womb. I could trust him; he is my God, my Rock, my Shelter, and he loves me more than I love myself. He doesn't send a thirsty soul to a dry well. He would fulfill me in his time and his way. —Danette

"THE ONLY THING I'VE BEEN POURING OUT IS MY HEART, POURING IT OUT TO GOD. DON'T FOR A MINUTE THINK I'M A BAD WOMAN. IT'S BECAUSE I'M SO DESPERATELY UNHAPPY AND IN SUCH PAIN THAT I'VE STAYED HERE SO LONG." ELI ANSWERED [HANNAH], "GO IN PEACE. AND MAY THE GOD OF ISRAEL GIVE YOU WHAT YOU HAVE ASKED OF HIM." "THINK WELL OF ME—AND PRAY FOR ME!" SHE SAID, AND WENT HER WAY. THEN SHE ATE HEARTILY, HER FACE RADIANT.
—1 Samuel 1:16–18 *The Message*

Shannon's Journal

Dear God,

I write in my promise book all the things I feel you're telling me. When I felt you say it was time to try again, I'd take a step toward a treatment and watch and listen. If money came pouring in, or I saw you opening doors for schedules or appointments or tests, I felt that was a sign to proceed. If house repairs came by the dozen, I'd hold back. Now, I didn't always gracefully accept these delays. I cried and prayed when house repairs required thousands of dollars. All I could see was IVF money going out the window, and I didn't see where new money would come from.

I'm also learning age is a huge factor in getting pregnant, and it will be much harder after I'm thirty-five. We'll have to be flexible with our future plans. It looks like we could be raising kids later in life then we expected. We're not giving up, God. Are you asking us to consider adoption? Where should we put our resources to give us the best chance at having another child?

We're weighing our options, and Dan's ready to try adoption. I'm not so sure. We had our first meeting with the adoption group at Saddleback, and God, it was so painful. Every moment I felt the hurt building up . . . God, I know you know my heart's desires. I ache to feel a baby in my belly again, the kicks, the movements, the sensation of his or her presence.
Longingly, Shannon

Two Mommies-in-Waiting Share

After all the injections and implantation of three embryos, we knew God answered our prayers as we cradled our miracle baby. We thanked God for the blessing of a beautiful, healthy child! Six months later, we began trying for a second child. This time God spared me the infertility treatment ordeal; I conceived naturally and gave birth to our second gift from God. Our third bundle of joy completed our family, we thought. Two and a half years later, God blessed us with our fourth child.

In looking back over the past seven years, I'm awestruck over God's goodness, mercy, and timing. Despite my temper tantrums and angry accusations during the initial infertility and our late start at becoming parents, God graciously granted my heart's desire for children four times! I'm also mindful of the lessons the Lord taught me: God is sovereign and doesn't owe me anything, including children. He's not a "genie in a bottle" to be commanded at will. He sometimes requires his children to take a difficult or risky step of faith before he provides a solution. As nightmarish as this trial was, it birthed a beautiful faith along with precious children. —Kelly

Shortly after giving our infertility heartache over to the Lord, the Bible study I was attending studied the day before Jesus' crucifixion in Matthew 26. Suddenly everything clicked. God, in Jesus, understands feeling abandoned by those closest to you. He knows what it means to have difficulty with his sovereign will, but he desires for us to ask for it in our lives anyway because his plan is much bigger than our own, and he will conform our will to his if we ask.

God said to me, "I understand." I felt God was answering my prayers as to when we should start trying for a baby again. Two weeks later, I found out I was pregnant. I'm now at twenty-one weeks as I write this. I'd never made it past week eight before. We're having a son named Gabriel Neihl. We hope for our angel to be a messenger of God's good news of hope to a hurting world someday. —Michele

Janet's Mentoring Moment

Kelly and Michele now see what God was up to and the lessons they learned, but during the trials, their hearts railed at God. Kim, Shannon, and all the in-waiting couples also saw God's plan and timing work out perfectly when they surrendered their will to his will. But they didn't recognize or appreciate this until *after* he revealed the end of a story they hadn't written for themselves. For those who held a baby in their arms, they applauded his rewrite; for those who didn't, they accepted their roles in his new script for them.

Today's obstacles may be God's rewrites. If you're in a place of worry and frustration and God seems distant, rest assured he isn't. He just writes with a different pen and wears a different watch than you do.

God's Love Letter to You

Dear_____ and_____,

Elkanah slept with Hannah his wife, and I, God, began making the necessary arrangements in response to what she had asked. Before the year was out, Hannah had conceived and given birth to a son. She named him Samuel, explaining, "I asked God for him" (1 Sam. 1:19–20 *The Message*, paraphrased).
Author of life, God

Couple's Prayer

Precious Heavenly Father, We are grateful that you, God, made our life complete when we placed all the pieces before you. When we got our act together, you gave us a fresh start. Now we're alert to your ways; we don't take you for granted. Every day we review the ways you work; we try not to miss a trick. We feel put back together, and we're watching our step. God, you rewrote the text of our lives when we opened the book of our hearts to your eyes. Amen (Ps. 18:20–24 *The Message,* paraphrased).

Your Letter to God

List ten ways you've seen God work in your life. How does this list help you rely on God in your current situation?

Dear God, _____ *Date:* _____

_____

_____

_____

_____

_____

_____

_____

_____

_____

_____

_____

_____

_____

_____

_____

_____

_____

_____

_____

Chapter Nineteen

PRAYING EXPECTANTLY

BEFORE I FORMED YOU IN THE WOMB I KNEW YOU,
before you were born I set you apart.
—Jeremiah 1:5

Petitioning God

It was such a surprise when we found out we were expecting twins and maybe triplets. But my dreams plummeted when the next blood test resulted in a much lower hCG, and we feared the worst. After calling my mom and her wonderful prayer chain, we held our breath and waited on the Lord. One baby survived. —Mandy

WE CONSTANTLY PRAY FOR YOU, THAT OUR GOD MAY COUNT YOU WORTHY OF HIS CALLING, AND THAT BY HIS POWER HE MAY FULFILL EVERY GOOD PURPOSE OF YOURS AND EVERY ACT PROMPTED BY YOUR FAITH.
—2 Thessalonians 1:11

Kim's Journal

Dear God,
I just learned that my mom and Dave have been fasting from sweets and desserts and praying to you that Shannon and Dan and Toby and I would become parents. They kept fasting and praying for us even after Shannon and Dan had Josh. Wow, that's a huge sacrifice. I feel a little guilty, though, that they're more dedicated and steadfast in praying for us than we are. They're giving up something while we go about our lives. I know they really love us, God, to make a sacrifice—just like you sacrificed your only Son for us. I guess I see it as my parents suffering right along with us, and that gives me so much comfort.
Gratefully, Kim

A Mommy-in-Waiting Shares

I'd been praying for a baby: the deepest desire of my heart, second only to my husband's salvation. When I was told I'd probably never have a child of my own, I cried out to the Lord: *If I wasn't meant to be a mom, why have I had to go through this month-to-month heartache? Why, Lord?* Then I realized that after a twenty-year rebellion, I'd recommitted my life to the Lord and given him my marriage, my unbelieving husband, and my future: everything except this desire for a baby. I began praying a new prayer: *Lord, I still want to be a mom and believe that Russ and I would be great parents. But I want your will more than anything. So, Lord, I pray that you will either let me have a baby or give me peace about not having one.*

God answered my prayers for peace. I'm not a mom. But I *am* a proud aunt. I *am* the honorary grandmother of my niece's son. I *am* a frequent storyteller to the little ones at church. —Sauni

Janet's Mentoring Moment

One Easter dinner at our house, during Kim's and Shannon's infertility struggles, the evening's discussion revolved solely around fertility treatments. I felt the Lord's prompting for my husband Dave and me to lay hands on and pray over each couple. We didn't pray for them to get pregnant, because we weren't sure if that was God's plan, but we did petition him to allow each couple to become parents.

Later that week, I felt the Lord's prompting: *How badly do you want your daughters to become mothers?* Badly! Dave and I decided to pray and fast from sugar and sweets daily until both couples were parents. We didn't tell anyone what we were doing: it was a commitment between the Lord and us. Shannon became pregnant five months later with Josh, and I'll save Kim's story for later, but God did hear our petitions.

Melissa confessed she felt guilty when her Bible study class was praying for her because she didn't think her situation "qualified," since she and her husband had *only* been trying to get pregnant for two years. She heard a radio interview with Drew Cline, a Christian recording artist and former lead singer for NewSong, and it had taken his wife and him eight years to have a baby, which seemed more worthy of prayer to Melissa. "Eight years, now that's a lot of praying!" she said.

Your every need is important to God. He says, "Until now you have not asked for anything in my name. Ask and you will receive, and your joy will be complete" (John 16:24). Start asking him, and ask everyone you know to start asking. Telling people specifically how to pray for you enlists an army of prayer warriors flooding the heavens. God may not answer in the way you expected, but he will answer whether one, two, or hundreds are praying.

God's Love Letter to You

Dear_____ and_____,

Take this most seriously: A yes on earth is yes in heaven; a no on earth is no in heaven. What you say to one another is eternal. I mean this. When two of you get together on anything at all on earth and make a prayer of it, I, your Father in heaven, go into action. And when two or three of you are together because of me, you can be sure that I'll be there (Matt. 18:18-20 *The Message,* paraphrased).

Hearing your petitions, God

Couple's Prayer

Lord, Help us be bold and specific in asking for prayer and believing that you, Father, hear us and will answer. Sometimes we don't want to tell people about our infertility, and yet we know that shortens the list of people praying. Help us remember to pray for our support groups and friends. Let us never tire of praying, even when we don't see immediate answers. Amen.

PRAYING PERSISTENTLY

Now for the fun part: waiting and, yes, more praying. I was praying for a healthy unborn baby. I prayed for the birth mom to make wise and healthy choices. I prayed believing God, believing he had a baby chosen, hand-picked especially for us, an infant growing inside of a womb. It's weird being an adoptive mom-in-waiting. You wonder just like any expectant mother: What will our baby look like? What color eyes or hair? Will it be a boy or a girl? Lord, what kind of child have you chosen for me? —Cindy

PRAY CONTINUALLY.
—1 Thessalonians 5:17

Shannon's Journal

Dear God,

A major source of my hope came from *The Power of Prayer (One Minute Devotions)* by E. M. Bounds that I got on my thirty-fifth birthday because I felt blue we hadn't had a second baby. This devotional was all about persistent prayer and how you, God, want us to keep asking and

asking because prayer draws us nearer to you. I dwelt on these devotions, and each day they gave me encouragement to keep praying and talking to you about my infertility issues.
Persistently praying, Shannon

A Mommy-in-Waiting Shares

Heather shares a time of persistent, conversational prayer with God:

> Heather: God, you already know my desire. I've told you a thousand times.
>
> God: *Yes, but is that unfulfilled desire stopping you from really experiencing me? Lavishing on me? Loving me? Will you give over this dream?*
>
> Heather: God, what are you talking about? (frustrated) God, you have my everything. I love you. I live every breath for you. You have it all!
>
> God: *What about your desire to have children? That journey.*
>
> Heather: (mad) The journey of not feeling loved by you? Abandoned? The journey of feeling how you are late on this one, God? The journey of Mark and I dedicating our hearts and lives to you, serving you, planning and praying for three years? The journey of not being able to start a family and the overwhelmingly painful desire to be a mom? That journey?
>
> God: *Yes.*

Then I realize he wants every piece of my heart . . . the uncertainty, the fear, the anger, the parts I don't want to admit to. It all belongs to him, and allowing him to have control over those painful areas is a way to love and lavish God!

> Heather: OK, God . . . I will allow you to hold me. I'll lean on you in this.
>
> God: *No.*
>
> Heather: No?
>
> God: *I will CARRY YOU!*

And I know he will!

Janet's Mentoring Moment

Persistent prayer helps resist doubt and restores faith that God can and will answer you according to his Word. Many of our cries to God are more to convince ourselves, not him, that he'll meet all our needs. Worship, prayer, and reading God's Word remind us of his unfailing power and love for us. Throughout this book, you've been personalizing and praying Scripture. Praying God's Word back to him is one way to know you're praying God's will.

God's Love Letter to You

Dear_____ and_____,

The Holy Spirit helps you in your weakness. For example, you don't know what I, God, want you to pray for. But the Holy Spirit prays for you with groanings that cannot be expressed in words. And I, the Father, who knows all hearts knows what the Spirit is saying, for the Spirit pleads for you believers in harmony with my own will (Rom. 8:26–27 NLT, paraphrased).
Prayerfully yours, God

Couple's Prayer

Oh Lord, We keep praying to you, Lord, hoping this time you will show us favor. In your unfailing love, O God, answer our prayer with your sure salvation. Amen. (Ps. 69:13 NLT, paraphrased)

GOD ALWAYS ANSWERS PRAYERS

Prayer isn't answered in our time, but God's time.
And God never makes a mistake. —Lisa J.

The Lord has heard my weeping. The Lord has heard my plea; the
Lord will answer my prayer.
— Psalm 6:8–9 NLT

Kim's Journal

Dear God,
After the worst Christmas of my life with all my siblings having children, Toby and I anxiously awaited "the call" that a birth mom had picked us. So many unknowns. It's not like being pregnant, counting the weeks and days before your due date. It could happen any day, or it could be years away.

One day as I was praying, I felt an overwhelming sense to pray specifically that if you wanted us to adopt a baby, it would happen quickly. After not having a period or ovulating for over three years, my period had started coming regularly. I felt I might get pregnant soon, and if I did, our adoption agency would put our case on hold to reopen later if we chose.

Daily I prayed for a quick adoption. Then the morning of January 12, about a month and a half after submitting our profile, we received a call that a birth mom had chosen us! Her baby was born January 9 and was full Hispanic, but they didn't know if it was a boy or girl. The birth mom was fifteen years old and in denial she was pregnant, so she hadn't had prenatal care, but the baby was healthy and passed all the newborn tests. Since the birthmother didn't have a prearranged adoption plan, the baby went into interim care.

I said, "YES!" I wanted to move forward. They promised to call back with more information and set up a meeting with the birth mom. Hanging up the phone, I was hysterical. I was going to be a mom! Thank you, God! Thank you, thank you, thank you! You heard my prayers and answered them quickly.

Ironically, I started my period that same day. I thanked you that I wasn't pregnant.
Hysterically grateful, Kim

A Mommy-in-Waiting Shares

My rheumatologist warned, "If you want to have a baby, don't wait any longer. You're not going to get better." I had lived with rheumatoid arthritis (RA) since I was twenty-four. At twenty-eight and married two years, I went off my medications trying to get pregnant, but a year later my RA was flaring badly, and my husband and I decided to put the dream of conception aside and start the journey of adoption with Bethany Christian Services.

We had our fears that most adoptive parents deal with, such as a birth mom changing her mind, but we surrendered it all over to God. The irony was that after a year of doing everything in my power to become pregnant, suddenly I didn't want to become pregnant. Once I was back on my medications, including a mild form of injected chemotherapy, a healthy pregnancy would become unlikely. Friends would say, "Oh, you'll get pregnant. Just relax and it will happen. We'll pray for you." I tried to explain, "No! I don't want *it* to happen now!" No one quite knew how to pray for us.

We wanted prayers for an adoption, and after prayerfully waiting for two years, "the call" came. Two weeks later a beautiful baby boy arrived to a birth mom who had chosen us. At the hospital, following an adoption ceremony that included her family, she came over to give me a hug. "I trust you completely," she said, looking deeply into my eyes. *Why?* I wondered. *I have no idea what I'm doing.*
—Lisa Copen

Janet's Mentoring Moment

Initially, Kim's burning desire was to be pregnant and carry a child, and yet, like Lisa Copen, she found herself asking God not to let her get pregnant so she could adopt. God had broadened their hearts to embrace loving a baby who didn't come from their womb but who desperately needed a mommy and daddy—something neither woman would have expected when first starting their journey to parenthood. God changed their perspective and their petition to match his interests: "Orphans get parents" (Ps. 10:17 *The Message*).

God doesn't always answer prayer the way we expect. That's why it's important to pray as Jesus did, "Everything is possible for you. . . . Yet I want your will, not mine" (Mark 14:36 NLT). God looks at the overall, global picture, and *our* plans aren't always *his* plans. Our prayers often are motivated by *our* interests, but God answers with *his* interests. Pray your desires, but check to see if your desires focus on your interests or God's. When my husband and I were praying for Kim and Shannon, we didn't pray for them to get *pregnant*, we prayed for them to become *parents* in whatever way God chose.

An answer we don't like is still an answer. You praise God if a child comes. Can you praise him if it doesn't happen or doesn't happen the way you expected? Like Mommy-in-Waiting Sauni, Rachel L. prayed for peace if she wasn't going to have children, and God answered her prayers. Peace *is* possible, even when our deepest earthly desires go unmet, because we know God has eternal plans for us in the family of God.

Rachel L. wrote, "As I shifted from being obsessed with conceiving to laying it all in God's hands, I heard from God. With listening ears, I heard that Jesus Christ is a son and a brother to all of us. I thought about him linking up his Apostle John with his mother Mary as family, at the cross. In this temporary age, you may have the blessing of a quiver full of children in the biological sense, but there is a higher sense of family that will make up our eternal life. And Christ is the center of that family."

God's Love Letter to You

*Dear*_____ *and*_____ *,*

This is God, your God, speaking to you. Call for help when you're in trouble—I'll help you, and you'll honor me (Ps. 50:7b,15 *The Message*). All that's required is that you really believe and do not doubt in your heart. Listen to me! You can pray for anything, and if you believe, you will have it (Mark 11:23–24 NLT).

Answering prayers, God

Couple's Prayer

We prayed to the Lord, and he answered us, freeing us from all our fears. When we look to him for help, we will be radiant with joy; no shadow of shame will darken our faces. Amen (Ps. 34:4–5 NLT, paraphrased).

PRAISING GOD

I'm even grateful for our fertility challenges. Had it not been for infertility, Robert and I may have taken parenting for granted. Instead, we view every child as a gift and we treasure our [adopted] sons as surprise packages from God.[1] —Laura Christianson

Surrendering my will and wants to God's will and ways allowed me truly to praise him even when I had no hope of being a mom. —Robin

THE LORD IS MY STRENGTH AND MY SHIELD; MY HEART TRUSTS IN HIM, AND I AM HELPED. MY HEART LEAPS FOR JOY AND I WILL GIVE THANKS TO HIM IN SONG.
—Psalm 28:7

Kim's Journal

Dear God,

A friend took me shopping to pick up newborn necessities. I'd have a "welcome home" party instead of a shower after our baby was with us, but in the meantime, I needed diapers, bottles, onsies. . . .What an exciting shopping trip! I hadn't allowed myself to go down the baby aisle before because it was too painful. Now I was having the time of my life picking out baby items for *my* baby.

Brandon was two weeks old when he came home to be with us—his forever family. Picking him up at the interim family's house was the most exciting and scary thing I've ever done. When Toby and I arrived and saw him for the first time, I fell instantly in love. God, I knew he was the child you had envisioned for us long before he was born. He was perfect, with ten fingers and toes and a full head of jet-black, curly hair. The interim family was a retired couple, and this was their ministry. Brandon was their forty-third newborn.

This wonderful couple showed us how to prepare a bottle, bathe him, care for his umbilical stump, and diaper and dress him, and they let me feed and burp him. Oh God, I was so nervous; I had no idea how to do any of this. It was like a baby care 101 crash course. After we thanked them for all they had done for him and for teaching us how to care for him, we put

Brandon into his car seat and loaded him into the car for the two-hour ride back home. But we couldn't leave; we sat there in amazement that there was a baby in the backseat. *Our* baby! It was surreal: we drove to someone's house and left with a baby. We looked at each other and said in unison, "I can't believe they're letting us take this baby! What are we doing?"

We prayed before we drove away, "Thank you, God! You are so good and faithful! Thank you for entrusting us with this precious baby boy." I rode in the backseat on the way home so I could stare at his beautiful face and study his features. I called my mom and Dave, who had been fasting from sugar and sweets and praying for us to become parents and told them to go out and have a hot fudge sundae—we had our baby!

Praising, Kim

A Mommy-in-Waiting Shares

We wanted a big family. Married at nineteen, we started trying to have children after three years. I had surgeries to help the process, and after several years of infertility treatment, I finally became pregnant. At five months, I lost the baby and never got pregnant again. Then at age twenty-nine, I had a radical hysterectomy. I thought: *Why did God do this to me?* I experienced months of depression and problems in my job and home life.

We decided to apply for adoption through the county. I called their office monthly and was starting to give up, but something always brought me back. We prayed and prayed for six years before the call came that we had waited for day and night: Were we still interested in adoption? Yes! They had a three-year-old boy for us. We said if we had a boy we wanted to name him Christopher. When they said his name was Christopher, we knew God had answered our prayers. We praise God for our son Chris, the blessing of our life. —Lisa J.

Janet's Mentoring Moment

Much of the infertility journey entails pleading, begging, bargaining, cajoling, crying out to God, and praising him. Praising goes beyond thanking God because thanking implies you've received something you wanted. The true test of faith is when you praise him solely for who he is, regardless of whether you get what you want. He is a good and glorious God *all* the time. Use the Prayer & Praise Journal, page 272, to record praises to your Heavenly Father.

God's Love Letter to You

Shout your praises to me, everybody! Let loose and sing! Strike up the band (Ps. 98:4 *The Message*, paraphrased)!

Hearing your praises, God

Couple's Prayer

Father, We praise you even when we can't see your plan. You are worthy of our praise and our worship *all* the time. We love you, Lord. We cannot imagine going through this ordeal without you by our side. Thank you for your constant love and protection. Praise you from whom all blessings flow. Amen.

HE IS THE GOD OF MIRACLES

We believe the way we received our adopted baby is a miracle that shows how God's timing is completely perfect. God is a composer conducting a beautiful symphony, and only when every note is played with perfect timing (his timing), that's when it works. —Cindy

The miracle is best described this way: For twelve years our twin daughters were frozen as embryos in a fertility clinic waiting for us to become their family. —Ken and Karen

GOD CAN DO ANYTHING!
—Luke 1:37 NCV

Kim's Journal

Dear God,

You are amazing! The Miracle Worker. When that little pregnancy stick showed a "plus" sign, and my sweet little five-week-old baby boy was peacefully lying beside me, I became hysterical once again. I probably looked like a chicken running around the room as I laughed and cried, waving the stick in the air yelling, "God, you sure do have a sense of humor!" I couldn't believe this was actually happening. Now I had my baby *and* I was pregnant.

God, you didn't tell us "No." You just said, "Trust me." I can't imagine life without Brandon. I thank you every day for your love and faithfulness. You never left my side; you were with me always.

Seeing the big picture, Kim

A Mommy-in-Waiting Shares

God has blessed us in many ways through this experience, and we know he has a great plan for our beautiful adopted little girl, Savannah, who is now almost four. We've had many miracles bless our family in our walk of faith with Jesus. Savannah has brought into our lives love and countless experiences. All along, God's plan was for her to be in our family. She even looks like her handsome "Daddy." —Jackie

Janet's Mentoring Moment

Considering the intricacies of conception, *every* birth is a miracle. *Every* baby is amazing, no matter how he or she comes into your life. All children are God's children. Only God can create a baby, and only God can overcome impossibilities. There are no coincidences in a believer's life. God performs miracles. Anticipate them. Pray for them. Give God the glory.

The Christmas after Brandon's adoption and Katelyn's birth, I wrote a poem about God bringing Brandon into our family. Enjoy!

A HOME FOR BRANDON

Thompson Christmas Poem

> Two pregnant teenagers
>> One delivering in a stable in Bethlehem.
>> One delivering in a hospital in Stockton.
> Two babies born
>> One destined to save the world.
>> One destined to be saved from the world.
> Two acts of God
>> One womb divinely opened.
>> One womb divinely closed.
> Two miracles
>> One Immaculate Conception.
>> One omniscient selection.
> Two homeless children
>> One cradled in a lowly manger.
>> One cradled by a kind stranger.
> Two adoptive parents
>> One loved Jesus as his firstborn son.
>> One loved Brandon as their firstborn son.

Two little boys
> One gives eternal life.
> One given earthly life.

Two purposes
> One fulfilled God's plan for Earth.
> One fulfilled God's plan for Katelyn's birth.

Two Christmas stories
> One of hope, love, and joy.
> One of two precious gifts . . . a girl and a boy. ©2005

God's Love Letter to You

Dear_____and_____,

Jesus says to you, "With man this is impossible, but with God all things are possible" (Matt. 19:26, paraphrased).

The miracle maker's Son, Jesus

Couple's Prayer

Dearest Jesus, We're praying for a miracle. We thank you for all the miracles we've seen you do in our lives and for dying on the cross and rising from the dead to offer us the miracle of eternal life. Help us keep our eyes focused on you and the amazing things we see you do every day. Thank you, Jesus, for giving us the opportunity to experience miracles in this lifetime. Amen.

Your Letter to God

Does God impress something specific on your heart to pray for right now? Can you see his hand working in your life, maybe in a miracle or two? Praise God for your many blessings.

Dear God,_____Date:_____

Chapter Twenty

_____

_____

_____

_____

_____

_____

RESTORING THE JOY!

HALLELUJAH!
THANK GOD! PRAY TO HIM BY NAME!
TELL EVERYONE YOU MEET WHAT HE HAS DONE!
SING HIM SONGS, BELT OUT HYMNS,
TRANSLATE HIS WONDERS INTO MUSIC!
HONOR HIS HOLY NAME WITH HALLELUJAHS,
YOU WHO SEEK GOD. LIVE A HAPPY LIFE!
KEEP YOUR EYES OPEN FOR GOD, WATCH FOR HIS WORKS;
BE ALERT FOR SIGNS OF HIS PRESENCE.
—Psalm 105:1–4 *The Message*

A Transforming Blessing

Going through infertility was a blessing because of the growth in our relationship and understanding of each other, and the awareness of God's time vs. our time. We started praying more and relying on his control rather than ours. —Jackie

It's great how when you're really walking with God, you see the blessing in everything. What a lesson for me. —Karen

DON'T COPY THE BEHAVIOR AND CUSTOMS OF THIS WORLD, BUT LET GOD TRANSFORM YOU INTO A NEW PERSON BY CHANGING THE WAY YOU THINK. THEN YOU WILL LEARN TO KNOW GOD'S WILL FOR YOU, WHICH IS GOOD AND PLEASING AND PERFECT.
—Romans 12:2 NLT

Shannon's Journal

Dear God,
Trying to have another child has been a journey, such heartache we've endured. It's hard to walk away without having succeeded. I feel like it's very possible IVF could work again, yet I realize I'm too tired to try . . . too worn out from the process. I'm burnt out. I feel emotionally beaten down.

Yet I feel a big part of me has grown stronger. I now know nothing can destroy me when you're carrying me and I have you to come to. I have more faith, strength, and trust for having walked this path. I feel overwhelming sadness, but tomorrow is a new day. I'm tired of disappointment. I'm ready to have my second child and complete my family. I'm ready to move on. Too many sad times. I want off this rollercoaster. God, we're considering adoption—prepare our child's mom. Help her recognize us and us her.

Blessings, Shannon

A Mommy- and Daddy-in-Waiting Share

Not knowing at the time what God had in store for us, we were grieving at the thought of never having our own child, but now we're thankful we were unable to conceive. Odds are we never would have chosen this path on our own, but fostering has turned out to be a passion and purpose we both share. This journey of adopting Blake through fostering has been more awesome than we ever could have imagined. —Cindy and Donald

Janet's Mentoring Moment

Suffering transforms our character: we have a deeper level of maturity and understanding of God, others, and ourselves. Many couples referred to their infertility journey as a blessing and a gift as they discovered the wisdom and reasons behind God's perfect plan. They didn't enjoy infertility, but most agreed this experience changed their lives for the better. That might be difficult for you to consider right now. It was tough for them, too, as they went through treatments, procedures, processes, and decisions while praying, "Help, Lord!" "We're so sad, Lord." "Please give us a child!" However, as God's plan began unfolding, they finally appreciated why he had them on the infertility journey.

Don't worry if it's too soon to think positively about your infertility. Tuck these thoughts away in your mind and heart, and when the time is right, reread this section. Or, perhaps you're ready to say with the other couples: Lord, we wouldn't have chosen infertility, but thank you for the ways you've used it to mold and make us into godlier people. Every couple who surrendered their will to God's will realized a purpose in their infertility and rediscovered joy.

When Kim and Toby heard Bruce Wilkinson speak at church that day, they took his challenge to surrender their "little dream" to God's Big Dream. How about you? Wilkinson says, "Therefore, you need to make a decision. Will you give God permission to do His work—for as long as He wants, in the ways that He wants, to change you as deeply as He wants—to prepare you for your Big Dream? It's a huge commitment, but your Dream is worth it. And your decision will open the door to joy in the midst of any circumstance."[1]

I pray someday you'll see you aren't the person you were before infertility touched your life and God transformed your heart and prepared you for his Big Dream.

God's Love Letter to You

Dear_____and_____,

My thoughts are completely different from yours, and my ways are far beyond anything you could imagine. For just as the heavens are higher than the earth, so are my ways higher than your ways and my thoughts higher than your thoughts. I send out my word, and it always produces fruit. It will accomplish all I want it to, and it will prosper everywhere I send it. You will live in joy and peace. The mountains and hills will burst into song, and the trees of the field will clap their hands! (Isa. 55:8–9, 11–12 NLT, paraphrased)

Transformer of lives, God

Couple's Prayer

Lord, Transform us and make us into the people you designed us to be. This isn't a journey we would have chosen for ourselves, but now that we're on it, please help us acknowledge the blessings and become better, not bitter. Show us your Big Dream for us. Amen.

IT FEELS GOOD BEING HAPPY!

Our boys joined our family through embryo adoption. I like to tell people that I gave birth to my adopted kids! —Julie

A HAPPY HEART MAKES THE FACE CHEERFUL,
BUT HEARTACHE CRUSHES THE SPIRIT.
—Proverbs 15:13

Shannon's Journal

Dear God,

Well, I don't sweat the small stuff anymore. If Dan doesn't have a job or is in danger of losing one, I don't worry as much because I've watched you come through and take care of us many times over. If I have to move or lose my house or keep driving our old car, it doesn't bother

me because I know how important my family is in comparison. Any obstacle that looks insur-
mountable, I just say, "That's OK because I've got my family and that's all I need." I want to live
happier days not carrying around this hurt and loss.
Choosing joy, Shannon

A Mommy-in-Waiting Shares

Now we understand the wisdom of why we couldn't have children, because we
have the one child God created just for us, and our adopted son Mark has the parents God created for him. We'll never know how bitter the road would have been
had we pursued paths on our own. We just know the incredible sweetness of the
last seventeen years. We don't know why God chose to do it this way. We're just
grateful he did. —Robin and Ray

Janet's Mentoring Moment

"Those who sow in tears will reap with songs of joy" (Ps. 126:5). You may not be
at a point where you're feeling happy, but find solace in knowing that God and his
Word can help you live a joyful life while you wait on his promise. Whatever way
God chooses to fulfill your dream, you will know inexplicable joy a fertile husband
and wife would never experience. Until then, join in with God's people who say:
My joy is in you, Lord. My hope is in you, Lord.

God's Love Letter to You

Dear_____ and_____,
May I, the God of hope, fill you with all joy and peace as you trust in me, so that you may over-
flow with hope by the power of the Holy Spirit (Rom. 15:13, paraphrased).
Your restorer of joy, God

Couple's Prayer

Oh Father, We've been sad for so long, and we crave some happiness and joy in our lives. We
know there are good things happening for which we could rejoice, but they've been overshad-
owed by the deep loss and frustration shrouding everything. Help us release our sorrow to you
and embrace the good things you so graciously give us—the most important being our relationships with you and with each other. We're ready for a new outlook on life. Help us see our
world through your eyes. Amen.

YOU CAN REJOICE IN THE TRIALS

Get healthy, forgive, forget, find your true path: the only real way to be happy! Otherwise, you will spend a lot of time pouting and feeling sorry for yourself. —Karen

GOD WILL LET YOU LAUGH AGAIN;
YOU'LL RAISE THE ROOF WITH SHOUTS OF JOY.
—Job 8:21 *The Message*

Shannon's Journal

Dear God,

God, when I think back to the character traits I wrote down two years ago of the woman I wanted to become, I had no idea I'd have to walk through so much pain to get there. They just sounded like good things to work on in my spiritual life. I can't believe the ways I've stretched and grown. Everything I held on to is gone. Ego stripped away; the self I knew, gone. Lord, this journal chronicles our journey through infertility: we've had four pregnancies, three losses, and a tubal. I hope, dear God, that's not the end of our story. I hope you have a sibling for Josh, and we get to be parents again.

God, there's so much you have for us, things I cannot see and only sense are on the way. So much good, I feel it. I dreamt that I was pregnant and giving birth to a blue-eyed baby girl. Is this you? Are you speaking to me? Is this a promise I should hold on to? Will I be pregnant again? God, I'd love to experience your miracles and your wonders.

Now we're considering another round of IVF. I'm weighing so many things, and I ask for your wisdom and guidance. Speak to Dan and me. Lead us.

Dreaming again, Shannon

A Mommy- and Daddy-in-Waiting Share

We have three wonderful kids: our two heaven-sent adopted children—who are such a natural extension of our lives—and then, in our early forties and shortly after our sixteenth anniversary, in his perfect timing God blessed us with the natural pregnancy Gay Lynne always had desired. The blessing didn't come from pursuing Gay Lynne's desires but as a gift from the One she had learned to love even when it seemed his hand was against us. Now that the pain and suffering from years of infertility are a distant memory, we understand that God was "for us" all the time. We would gladly go through infertility again to experience the joy we have today with these amazing children. —Gay Lynne and Dan

Janet's Mentoring Moment

Have you had difficulty rejoicing in this infertility trial? Do the hardships far outweigh the blessings at this point? If so, I'm so sorry; I understand and so does God. Pray for comfort that the world cannot give. Let God wrap his arms around your heart and cheer you up. As blessings begin to unveil, thank God and write them down so you remember his faithfulness through all generations.

At the end of this chapter, there's a page titled "I Am So Happy Because . . ." It's a place to linger awhile and literally count your blessings. If you have trouble getting started, try beginning with gratitude for *today's* gift of life. As you write, your heart will begin singing, and you, too, will say, "I can rejoice in my trials." On difficult days, return to this page and read what you wrote.

God's Love Letter to You

Dear_____ and_____,
There, in my presence, you and your families shall eat and shall rejoice in everything you have put your hand to, because I, the LORD your God, have blessed you (Deut. 12:7, paraphrased).
Blessings, God

Couple's Prayer

Oh Lord, For you make us glad by your deeds, O LORD; we sing for joy at the works of your hands. How great are your works, O LORD, how profound your thoughts! Amen (Ps. 92:4–5, paraphrased).

Your Letter to God

Ask God to remind you of something that puts a smile on your face, restores joy, and shows you the light at the end of the tunnel.

Dear God,_____   Date:_____

_____

_____

_____

_____

I AM SO HAPPY BECAUSE . . .

I Have Things to Be Grateful For

I Have Many Blessings

Chapter Twenty-One

ENDING AT THE BEGINNING

"HE WILL REMOVE ALL OF THEIR SORROWS, AND THERE WILL
BE NO MORE DEATH OR SORROW OR CRYING OR PAIN. FOR
THE OLD WORLD AND ITS EVILS ARE GONE FOREVER.
AND THE ONE SITTING ON THE THRONE SAID,
"LOOK, I AM MAKING ALL THINGS NEW!"
AND THEN HE SAID TO ME, "WRITE THIS DOWN, FOR WHAT I TELL YOU IS
TRUSTWORTHY AND TRUE." AND HE ALSO SAID, "IT IS FINISHED!
I AM THE ALPHA AND THE OMEGA—THE BEGINNING AND THE END.
TO ALL WHO ARE THIRSTY I WILL GIVE THE SPRINGS
OF THE WATER OF LIFE WITHOUT CHARGE!"
—Revelation 21:4–6 NLT

Making Your Story Your Testimony

When I'm on the other side of infertility and you prove faithful, then I'll have this great testimony. God answered, "It is the journey that I have you on that is your testimony."
—Heather

Only God can make a baby. This realization has impacted the way I value life. Every child was a purposeful, planned creation of God. —Julie

GENERATION AFTER GENERATION STANDS IN AWE OF YOUR WORK; EACH ONE TELLS STORIES
OF YOUR MIGHTY ACTS.
—Psalm 145:4 *The Message*

Kim's Journal

Dear God,
Apparently you allowed us to conceive our daughter Katelyn the night before we picked up
Brandon from the interim family's house. God, people have had many things to say about our

situation, one being that we got pregnant because we took our mind off it and relaxed. I'm not sure if that's true, but the way I see it, you planned for Brandon to be our child, and if we'd gotten pregnant when we were trying so hard to fulfill *our* plan to become parents, we would have missed out on knowing and loving our son—we would have missed out on your Big Dream for us.

As we tell our story, people often respond, "That happens *all* the time." We assure them it doesn't; you just hear about it when it does. Many people adopt children but never conceive on their own. We advise prospective parents *not* to go into adoption thinking this will be their ticket to what their heart *really* desires—getting pregnant. We had grieved that loss. Getting pregnant wasn't a thought for us anymore, so we know everything was *all* part of your Master Plan for Brandon to have a forever home with us.

Brandon and Katelyn are only nine months and three days apart, so they kept us busy, and then you surprised us again when I got pregnant with Sienna! Now we *really* have a story to tell of a triple blessing beyond our wildest expectations: three babies within three years!
A mommy at last and lovin' it, Kim

Mommies- and Daddies-in-Waiting Share

My husband had faith that this experience of secondary infertility and miscarriages was part of God's design for a testimony we would someday share with others in similar situations. Through this journey, I've discovered that people who put their children up for adoption love them very much and are incredibly brave. God also has taught me to live in anticipation of trials. He uses them to prepare me for greater service, ministry, and joy and to test the validity of my faith. Most importantly, I've learned that when I don't understand what God is doing, he's still there. —Alice

Through embryo adoption, the Lord fulfilled Psalm 113:9 for me. My heart is now settled and full to overflowing. I am the grateful mother of two sets of twin girls. This is a new chapter to our infertility story. God delights in going above and beyond. It should not surprise us though: he is an awesome God. He has blessed us richly. Looking back at this journey, I see how he walked us through every step. I believe the answer to the question, "Dear God, why can't I have a baby?" is in the faces of our four beautiful daughters. The journey to this end has taken us through some great valleys and rocky terrain, but as someone once said, "Don't complain about being in the valley, it's where the best fertilizer is." In those valleys, God was working his character and purpose into our lives. He has strengthened our faith and fulfilled our hope. However, even if he hadn't answered our prayer for children, he would still be a great God, for it's who he is, not what he does or doesn't do, that we can count on. Jeff and I know that God chose us to travel this road and to share our story with others for whatever encouragement and hope it can bring, but mostly to honor God. He is faithful. He is good, and his mercies are new every morning. Trust his purpose in your life; he will amaze you! —Danette and Jeff

While working for KSLR Radio, a Christian station in San Antonio, Texas, I emceed a pro-life event where I reiterated that Christians are prepared to adopt children being sent to their deaths by abortion, and we're prepared to adopt children born out of wedlock. I added, "On a personal level, Amy and I ache to hold and raise a baby to be a champion for Jesus Christ. We would love to adopt." Providentially, after the event concluded, a friend in the audience approached Amy. "Is it really true you and Adam would be open to adoption?" "Absolutely!" Amy said. Our friend continued. "The daughter of a friend of mine is pregnant. She's eighteen, isn't married, and I think she's open to placing her child for adoption." With pregnant anticipation, Amy exclaimed, "What? Are you serious? Let me talk to Adam." —Adam McManus

Our story already is touching lives, and we want to give glory to God for the beginning of our adopted daughter Savannah's wonderful life. Please pass our story on to provide hope and encouragement to keep the faith. One wonderful outcome to all of this is the beautiful testimonies we share with so many other women who have battled this emotional rollercoaster called *infertility*. —Jackie

Janet's Mentoring Moment

Kim, Shannon, and the couples in this book shared their stories to offer you hope and encouragement. Each *story* became a *testimony* when God received the glory—the focus shifted from their pain to God's gain—regardless of how the story ended.

Daddy-in-Waiting Adam McManus, a Christian radio talk show host, used his platform to encourage adoption while expressing Amy's and his willingness to adopt after experiencing an ectopic pregnancy and miscarrying identical twins. The blessing for their transparency and vulnerability while furthering God's kingdom work was the adoption of their son, Honor.

Maybe you've heard "Make your mess your message." If life's too messy right now to see the message, follow the advice that Anissa gave to her sister and brother-in-law, Ben and Joanna, at the funeral of their twelve-day-old daughter, Grace, which was the third infant they had buried along with two miscarriages.

> Over the next few weeks and months, the verses you have known all your life may not seem to fit, nor bring the comfort you think they should. And that's OK. It doesn't mean you don't love God, or you don't have faith. Right now, you want baby Grace in your arms more than you want any lesson you're supposed to learn from this. You want her more than the lives that are being touched as a result of what you're going through. Give yourself permission not to have a testimony on your tongue. Give yourself permission to grieve for however long it takes.

When you're ready, God wants to use your testimony to change lives—starting with your own. These words are from Laura T., Gay Lynne's sister, whose own baby was born with Down syndrome while Gay Lynne was struggling with infertility.

> God builds our testimonies through our experiences . . . good or bad, and can use us to encourage others who are in the midst of similar circumstances. This still is no consolation for someone in the middle of the pain. Everyone who is a child of God will have a story to tell of some trial or difficulty that God has allowed, in order for him or her to develop into a more beautiful person. My sister, Gay Lynne, knows that now. She tells her story with joy. The pieces all are going together. God's ways are perfect. You don't see it then, only later after you've opened up your clenched fists to his will and say with Job, "Even though you slay me, yet I will trust you." (Job 13:15 NKJV, paraphrased)

Your testimony isn't how you did or didn't get a child; your testimony is how Jesus worked in your life on the infertility journey. A pastor friend of ours states this truth beautifully: "A changed life coupled to a clear testimony will attract people to Jesus; and in the end, that's what our life as a Christian is all about."

God's Love Letter to You

Dear_____and_____,

You're here to be light, bringing out the God-colors in the world. I, God, am not a secret to be kept. We're going public with this, as public as a city on a hill. If I make you light-bearers, you don't think I'm going to hide you under a bucket, do you? I'm putting you on a light stand. Now that I've put you there on a hilltop, on a light stand—shine! Keep open house; be generous with your lives. By opening up to others, you'll prompt people to open up with me, God, a generous Father in heaven. (Matt. 5:14–16 *The Message,* paraphrased)

Giving you a testimony, God

Couple's Prayer

Father, Please give us courage to tell our story in a way that spotlights you and not us. It's difficult reliving the pain or talking about the current struggles, but we know there are others who need to know they don't have to go through this infertility journey alone. You want to guide and lead them. Help us turn our story into our testimony. Amen.

THE END OF ONE JOURNEY IS THE BEGINNING OF THE NEXT

I'm not sure what we would choose in life if God showed the ending to us first. We don't know what is best for us. God does. —Simon

Everything will work out in the end. If it's not working out, it's not the end.[1] —Max Lucado

REMEMBER THE FORMER THINGS, THOSE OF LONG AGO; I AM GOD, AND THERE IS NO OTHER; I AM GOD, AND THERE IS NONE LIKE ME. I MAKE KNOWN THE END FROM THE BEGINNING, FROM ANCIENT TIMES, WHAT IS STILL TO COME. I SAY: MY PURPOSE WILL STAND, AND I WILL DO ALL THAT I PLEASE.
—Isaiah 46:9–10

Shannon's Journal

Dear God,

While we were waiting for a birthmother to choose us, Dan got a new job, and their insurance covers IVF! We felt that was confirmation to try again. Our fertility specialist, Dr. Werlin, recommended genetics testing first. While I wanted answers from those tests, I only had money to spend on one thing . . . testing or IVF. Talking to the doctor, I had a deep conviction that we just needed to do IVF one more time. To each concern he presented, I repeated my conviction. We took a risk and didn't do any further testing.

My cycle happened to coordinate with my doctors' schedules, and within a month, I had a laparoscopy and started the IVF hormones. We implanted the only three good embryos we had. Our first hCG levels were the lowest ever, and I thought for sure we would have another miscarriage. I had hoped for more than one embryo to attach with high levels. I thought starting with more embryos would be a guarantee at least one would make it. You wanted me to trust you, not a number.

Who would've thought thirty-five would be my best year ever?! We are twenty weeks' pregnant and having a girl. You've given us our dream, and I can't thank you enough for this gift. Our spirits were breaking, and you renewed our joy! Truly another miracle. I love feeling her move and grow. It's amazing. Thank you for this blessing. I pray for her health and for my body to support and nourish her until she's ready to be born.

Beginning again, Shannon

A Mommy- and Daddy-in-Waiting Share

The doctor implanted three fertilized eggs, and to our surprise, I became pregnant with triplets! At twenty-seven weeks, all three babies were born, tiny but beautiful! They were on ventilators in NICU, and it broke our hearts when Michael died at five days old. Prior to our children's third birthday, I conceived naturally with a healthy, full-term baby boy! After all we'd been through, we figured we couldn't get pregnant on our own, but we did!

I'm getting older and couldn't go through another multiple birth pregnancy, so our infertility specialist gave us information about the Snowflakes Frozen Embryo Adoption & Donation Program for our remaining frozen embryos. We were excited to help another infertile couple realize their dreams of having a family. We also wanted our pre-children raised by loving, supportive parents with values similar to ours. We didn't want our embryos, fertilized forms of life, thrown away or destroyed. It wasn't an easy decision to give our embryos up for adoption, but we know in our hearts it was the right thing to give life a chance and to give hope to another couple like ourselves. —Jennifer and Joe

Janet's Mentoring Moment

The end of Jennifer and Joe's infertility journey was the beginning of another couple's journey to becoming parents.

The end of Kim and Toby's infertility journey—opening their hearts and home to a sweet adopted baby boy and the surprise of two unexpected natural pregnancies—was the beginning of a crash course in parenting and raising three babies within three years, while championing the blessings of adoption.

The end of Shannon and Dan's infertility journey—one last try at IVF before adopting—was the beginning of opening their modest home to a teenage nephew in need of loving guidance, while also discovering God was opening Shannon's womb one more time for the precious baby girl their family prayed for. Jordan Ashley is our eleventh grandchild. Shannon says of Jordan, "I look at her and am still amazed; I'm reminded of how God worked in our lives in a big way. I trust Got a lot more."

Some couples chose to end the infertility journey without realizing a child and put their energies and efforts into beginning a ministry or serving God more fully. Verna and Mike decided to become foster parents, a decision Verna said, "Ended my obsession with becoming pregnant again, and began a time of freedom and joy that I haven't experienced in years. I actually could rejoice, instead of being angry, when a friend told me she was pregnant while 'barely trying'—something I hadn't been able to do in almost eight years. When I threw away the calendar of charting daily bodily functions, a burden lifted from my heart. There are so many children who need to experience a loving Christian home, why was I trying so hard to reproduce myself?"

Wherever you are on the journey—just beginning, feeling stuck in the middle, seeing your dreams fulfilled, or following a new dream—God is working on a parallel Dream that is bigger than you can imagine. It's never just about you; it's always about God's purpose of furthering his kingdom here on earth and taking care of *all* his children. He wants you to help him fulfill his vision while he works on helping you fulfill your dreams. Amy and Rick, who adopted out their frozen embryos, said the lesson they learned through the process was: "Our children are God's children. Perhaps they will have our DNA, but in an even more fundamental manner, they possess God's gift of life and the promise of eternity."

Jesus' death on the cross wasn't the end of the story God is writing. The cross was just the beginning, and because Jesus trusted God (I want your will, not mine—Mark 14:36), you and I have the opportunity to end our old, sinful life and begin a new life in Christ. The end of one journey is the beginning of the next adventure, and with God in your life, it will be a glorious one. Whatever you're going through, it will end well. Trust God for your new beginning. As C.S. Lewis writes:

> The things that began to happen after that were so great and beautiful that I cannot write them. And for us this is the end of all the stories, and we can most truly say that they all lived happily ever after. But for them it was only the beginning of the real story. All their life in this world and all their adventures in Narnia had only been the cover and the title page; now at last they were beginning Chapter One of the Great Story which no one on earth has read, which goes on for ever, in which every chapter is better than the one before.[2]

God's Love Letter to You
Dear_____ and_____,
My dear friends, I'm not writing anything new here. This is the oldest commandment in my book, and you've known it from day one. It's always been implicit in the Message you've heard from me. On the other hand, perhaps it is new, freshly minted as it is in both Christ and you—the darkness on its way out and the True Light already blazing (1 John 2:7–8 *The Message*, paraphrased)!
I AM the Alpha and the Omega, the Beginning and the End, the New Beginning, God

Couple's Prayer
Heavenly Father, Thank you for the new beginning you gave us when we accepted you into our hearts as our personal Savior. We know the end of our earthly life will be the beginning of our eternal life with you, but while you have us here, Father, use us for your glory. Let our journey and our lives draw others closer to you. We look forward with joy to our reunion with any of our lost little ones when our journey on earth ends, and our eternal life with you begins. Until then, let our lives be a testimony. Amen.

Your Letter to God
Have any of the stories you've read provided perspective on what God might want you to do? Is there a new dream to pursue or one to end? Talk with God about a new beginning. If you're ready to start a new life in Christ, go now to My New Beginning Prayer, page 245.

Dear God,   *Date:* _____

_____

_____

_____

_____

_____

_____

_____

_____

_____

AND THIS IS HIS PLAN: AT THE RIGHT TIME HE WILL BRING EVERYTHING
TOGETHER UNDER THE AUTHORITY OF CHRIST—EVERYTHING IN HEAVEN
AND ON EARTH. FURTHERMORE, BECAUSE OF CHRIST, WE HAVE RECEIVED AN
INHERITANCE FROM GOD, FOR HE CHOSE US FROM THE BEGINNING, AND ALL
THINGS HAPPEN JUST AS HE DECIDED LONG AGO.
—Ephesians 1:10–11 NLT

MY NEW BEGINNING PRAYER

Dear God,

I believe you sent your Son, Jesus, to die on a cross and rise to life three days later to wipe away my sins and give me eternal life with you. I know I have sinned, and I ask for your forgiveness. I don't understand everything about being a Christian, and I still have some questions, but I do know I want to accept you today into my heart, and I'm willing to learn more about what that means. Thank you for offering me the free gift of salvation. In Jesus' name, I pray. Amen!

Congratulations! You accepted Jesus into your heart as your personal Savior. Perhaps that was God's purpose and plan—his Big Dream—for your infertility journey.

Chapter Notes

Chapter One

1. Marlo Schalesky, *Empty Womb, Aching Heart* (Minneapolis: Bethany House, 2001), 11.
2. Excerpted from *The Adoption Decision*, Copyright 2007 by Laura Christianson, Published by Harvest House Publishers, Eugene, OR. Used by Permission. www.harvesthousepublishers.com, 75.
3. Christianson, *The Adoption Decision*, 75-76.
4. Ibid., 76.
5. Ibid., 76.
6. Judith C. Daniluk, Ph.D., *The Infertility Survival Guide* (Oakland, CA: New Harbinger Publications, Inc., 2001), 17.
7. Chris Adams, "My Struggle with Infertility: A Testimony from One Women's Leader," www.lifeway.com/article/151150.

Chapter Two

1. Heidi Schlumpf, "Inconceivable: The Spiritual Test of Infertility," *Marriage Partnership*, Summer 2007, 37.
2. Schlumpf, "Inconceivable," 38.
3. Ibid.
4. "Study: Acupuncture May Boost Pregnancy," *USA Today*, February 7, 2008, www.usatoday.com/news/health/2008-02-07-acupuncture-fertility_N.htm.
5. "Want a Baby? Hold the Fries," Health & Fitness, *The Orange County Register*, January 28, 2007, 3.
6. Linda Marsa, "Have You Gone Caffeine Crazy?" *Ladies' Home Journal*, June 2007, 156.
7. Schlumpf, "Inconceivable," 38.
8. Christianson, *The Adoption Decision*, 76.

Chapter Three

1. Christianson, *Adoption Decision*, 76-77.
2. Daniluk, *The Infertility Survival Guide*, 29–30.
3. Ginger Kolbaba and Christy Scannell, *Desperate Pastors' Wives* (New York: Howard Fiction, 2007), 39–40.

Chapter Four

1. "Infertility Tales," *Real Simple*, May 2007, 301.
2. Christianson, *The Adoption Decision*, 77.

Chapter Five

1. Christianson, *The Adoption Decision*, 89.

Chapter Seven

1. Christianson, *The Adoption Decision*, 77.
2. Daniluk, *The Infertility Survival Guide*, 63.

Chapter Ten

1.   Schlumpf, "Inconceivable," 40.
2.   Adams, "My Struggle with Infertility."
3.   Carla Drew, "A Sisterhood of Suffering," *Newsweek,* March 31, 2008, 20.
4.   Schlumpf, "Inconceivable," 40.

Chapter Eleven

1.   Karen Springen, "Love, Loss—And Love," *Newsweek,* December 3, 2007, 53.

Chapter Twelve

1.   Sue Hawkes, "The Baby Club," *Today's Christian Woman,* July/August 2007, 43.

Chapter Thirteen

1.   Max Lucado, *Fearless* (Nashville: Thomas Nelson, 2009), 7.
2.   Adams, "My Struggle with Infertility."

Chapter Fourteen

1.   Bob Perry, "When Mr. Fix-It Won't Do," *Marriage Partnership,* Summer 2007, 38–39.
2.   Christianson, *The Adoption Decision,* 78-80.
3.   Chris Tiegreen, *The One Year Walk with God Devotional* (Wheaton, IL: Tyndale House Publishers, Inc., 2004), August 14.

Chapter Fifteen

1.   Bruce Wilkinson, *The Dream Giver* (Colorado Springs: Multnomah Publishers, 2003), 114.
2.   Schlumpf, "Inconceivable," 40.
3.   Wilkinson, *The Dream Giver,* 113.

Chapter Eighteen

1.   Wilkinson, *The Dream Giver,* 133.
2.   Tiegreen, *One Year Walk with God,* July 24.

Chapter Nineteen

1.   Christianson, *The Adoption Decision,* 89.

Chapter Twenty

1.   Wilkinson, *The Dream Giver,* 121.

Chapter Twenty-One

1.   Lucado, *Fearless,* 160.
2.   C. S. Lewis, *The Last Battle* (New York: Collier Books, 1956), 183–184.

SANITY TOOLS

Glossary of Infertility Terms and Abbreviations

ART—assisted reproductive technologies

cerclage—stitching the cervix closed to prevent opening prematurely

D&C—dilation and curettage—a surgical procedure to remove contents of uterus, often performed after miscarriage

DI—donor insemination—using donated sperm

donor egg—using donated eggs

donor embryo—embryos produced and donated by another couple

EA—embryo adoption— adopting frozen embryos

ectopic pregnancy—embryo implants somewhere other than the uterus, usually in fallopian tube

EPT—early pregnancy test

endometriosis—endometrial tissue lining the uterus shed during menstruation, grows outside of the uterus

harvesting eggs—retrieval of eggs using a small needle inserted into the ovarian follicle following egg stimulation by hormone therapy

hCG—human chorionic gonadotropin—hormones produced by placenta, confirming pregnancy

HMO—Health Maintenance Organization—sets out guidelines under which doctors can operate. On average, costs less than comparable traditional health insurance, with a trade-off of limitations on the range of treatments available.

HSG—hysteropingogram—X-ray of fallopian tubes and uterus involving injection of dye into cervix

ICSI—intracytoplasmic sperm injection—variation of IVF—sperm is microinjected into eggs

IF—infertility

IUI—intrauterine insemination or artificial insemination—sperm injected through catheter into uterus

IVF—in vitro fertilization—fertilization of eggs in laboratory and embryos placed in uterus

laparoscopy—a scope is inserted through small incisions in abdomen to view abdominal cavity and reproductive organs

OB-GYN—obestetrician-gynocologist

OPK—ovulation predictor kit

PCOS—polycystic ovary syndrome—genetically linked hormonal imbalance preventing ovulation and possible overproduction of estrogen, thickening of the uterine lining, heavy and/or irregular periods

PGD—preimplantation genetic diagnosis—screening at-risk embryos before IVF implantation

PPO—Preferred Provider Option—a flexible health care option. The insurance company has a network of care providers to use at your discretion. The care provider files the claim with your PPO carrier, and you pay the difference between the bill and the insurance payment.

sonohysterogram—like the HSG but an ultrasound is used instead of X-rays

specialist in reproductive endocrinology and infertility—fertility specialist or infertility specialist

transfer—delicate placement of embryos near the middle of the endometrial cavity

TTC—trying to conceive

Note: This is not an exhaustive list but includes those used in this book. You can find additional terms and definitions online.

Research Notes

Source_____

Notes_____

_____

_____

_____

Source_____

Notes_____

_____

_____

_____

Source_____

Notes_____

_____

_____

Source_____

Notes_____

_____

_____

Source_____

Notes_____

_____

_____

Source_____

Notes_____

_____

_____

_____

National Contacts

Support and Information

American Fertility Association—National Office
666 Fifth Avenue, Suite 278   National Support Line   www.theafa.org
New York, NY 10103-0004   888-917-3777
A nonprofit organization with resources on both fertility treatments and adoption

A Place to Remember   1-800-631-0973   www.APlaceToRemember.com
A national clearinghouse of information for women facing complicated pregnancies, bed rest, or the death of a baby

Bed Rest Buddies   www.cafemom.com/group/108759

Charting Your Way to Conception
Free ovulation and fertility charts   www.fertilityfriend.com

Elizabeth Ministry   www.elizabethministry.com
Providing hope and healing for women and their families on issues related to childbearing, sexuality, and relationships

INCIID—The InterNational Council on Infertility Information Dissemination, Inc.
P.O. Box 6836   703-379-9178   www.inciid.org
Arlington, VA 22206   inciidinfo@inciid.org

In Due Season Ministries   www.indueseasonministries.org
A Virginia-based, non-profit 501(c)(3) organization which upholds Christian values and offers educational, mental, and spiritual support to women and men touched by infertility. The organization strives to increase awareness and implements health and wellness programs on a local, regional, and national basis.

M.E.N.D (Mommies Enduring Neonatal Death)
P.O. Box 1007   972-506-9000   www.mend.org
Coppell, TX 75019   Rebekah@mend.org
A Christian nonprofit organization with a bimonthly newsletter offering support to couples who have lost a baby in early pregnancy up to one year

RESOLVE National (not a Christian organization)
1310 Broadway   671-623-0744   www.resolve.org
Somerville, MA 02144-1779   info@resolve.org
Check for the local chapter in your area

Sidelines National Support Network   1-888-447-4754 (HI-RISK4)   www.sidelines.org
Based in Laguna Beach, California, a national volunteer network for women with pregnancy complications

The American Society for Reproductive Medicine (ASRM)
1209 Montgomery Highway   205-978-5000   www.asrm.com
Birmingham, AL 35216-2809

Adoption

Adoptive Families Magazine — www.adoptivefamilies.com

All God's Children International Adoption
1-800-214-6719 — www.allgodschildren.org

Bethany Christian Services   1-800-Bethany   www.bethany.org
Stepping Stones (quarterly newsletter)

Christian Adoption Services
Matthews-Mint Hill Road   704-847-0038   www.christianadopt.org
Matthews, NC 28105-1775   cas@christianadopt.org

National Adoption Center   1-800-862-3678   www.adopt.org
Helps place children in foster care with adoptive parents

National Council for Adoption   703-299-6633   www.adoptioncouncil.org
Member agencies in most states and a network of adoption services in over thirty countries

Nightlight Christian Adoptions—Domestic & International
714-693-5437 — www.nightlight.org

Scrapbooking   www.scrapbookmyadoption.com
www.scrapbookmyadoptionblog.com

Frozen Embryo Adoption and Donation

Snowflakes Frozen Embryo Adoption & Donation Program (through Nightlight)
4430 East Miraloma Avenue, Unit B   714-693-KIDS (5437)   www.snowflakes.org
Anaheim Hills, CA 92807   megan@nightlight.org
Note: Embryo adoption and donation can also be arranged through a private attorney

Fertility after Cancer

Fertile Hope
P.O. Box 624   889-994-HOPE   www.fertilehope.org
New York, NY 10014

Blogs

A Christian online forum   www.childlessnotbychoice.com

Adam McManus (A contributing Daddy-in-Waiting)   www.TakeAStand.net

Facebook

RESOLVE: The National Infertility Association

"Hannahs Hope" Seeking God's heart in the midst of infertility

In Due Season - Support for Those Touched by Infertility

Books and Resources
Infertile Couples Found Helpful

Spiritual Living

The Holy Bible
In the Meantime: The Practice of Proactive Waiting—Rob Brendle
The Power of Prayer (One Minute Devotions)—E.M. Bounds
The Dream Giver—Bruce Wilkinson
When Women Walk Alone: Finding Hope and Strength Through the Seasons of Life—Cindi McMenamin (www.StrengthForTheSoul.com, a contributing Mommy-in-Waiting)
A Sacred Sorrow: Meeting God in the Lost Language of Lament—Michael Card
The Hidden Face of God—Michael Card (musical CD)
Suffering and the Sovereignty of God—Edited by John Piper and Justin Taylor
Why? Trusting God When You Don't Understand—Anne Graham Lotz
Holding On to Hope: A Pathway through Suffering to the Heart of God—Nancy Guthrie
The Plan A Woman in a Plan B World—Debbie Taylor Williams
A Friend in the Storm—Cheryl Ricker (devotional)

Specific to Infertility and Loss of a Child

Trusting God Through Tears—Jehu Thomas Burton (a father's story)
Taking Charge of Your Fertility—Toni Weschler (non-Christian viewpoint, contains user-friendly explanation of women's health and monthly cycling)
The Infertility Companion—Christian Medical Association
The Infertility Survival Guide—Judith C. Daniluk, Ph.D. (informative, non-Christian viewpoint)
When the Cradle Is Empty: Answering Tough Questions About Infertility—John and Sylvia Van Regenmorter (editors of Bethany's *Stepping Stones* newsletter)
I'll Hold You in Heaven—Jack Hayford
Empty Womb, Aching Heart—Marlo Schalesky
Hannah's Hope: Seeking God's Heart in the Midst of Infertility, Miscarriage, & Adoption Loss—Jennifer Saake
Tender Fingerprints: A True Story of Loss and Resolution—Brad Stetson
Safe in the Arms of God: Truth from Heaven About the Death of a Child—John MacArthur
Miscarriage: A Man's Book—Rick Wheat
Moments for Couples Who Long for Children—Ginger Garrett (daily devotional)
Grieving the Child I Never Knew—Kathe Wunnenberg (devotional)

Adoption

The Adoption Decision: 15 Things You Want to Know Before Adopting—Laura Christianson (www.laurachristianson.com, a contributing Mommy-in-Waiting)
The Adoption Network: Your Guide to Starting a Support System—Laura Christianson
20 Things Adoptive Parents Need to Succeed—Sherrie Eldridge (www.sherrieeldridge.com)
Twenty Things Adopted Kids Wish Their Adoptive Parents Knew—Sherrie Eldridge
Forever Fingerprints . . . An Amazing Discovery for Adopted Children—Sherrie Eldridge
Questions Adoptees Are Asking—Sherrie Eldridge
The Making of Isaac Hunt—Linda Leigh Hargrove (fiction, www.llhargrove.com, a contributing Mommy-in-Waiting)

Making Decisions and Developing a Family Plan

You're continually faced with decisions and options. Prayerfully developing a plan in advance and establishing parameters you both agree on will alleviate anxiety and pressure later. Use the following questions to help formulate your plan *before* going beyond a point where you're no longer comfortable. Pray and discuss together your answers to the following:

- What are you both willing to sacrifice?
- Is your main goal to be biological parents or parents?
- How much money will you spend?
- Will you focus solely on conception?
- What time frame before considering other options?
- What doctor or clinic?
- What tests to have and avoid?
- What treatments?
- How many times to repeat procedures?
- Natural versus scientific intervention and what is the teaching of your faith?
- Is using donor sperm, eggs, or uterus to create life acceptable?
- Are you prepared to tell a child about his or her creation or adoption?
- Selecting only the genetically superior embryos or predetermining the sex?
- Freezing or destroying unused embryos or donating to science or another couple?
- Selective reduction of multiple pregnancies?
- Loving a child that doesn't have your blood and genes?
- Will you pursue adoption? Embryo adoption? Foster parenting?
- Adoption agencies or private adoption?
- Would you adopt a baby? Older child? Special needs? Different race?
- When will you say enough is enough?
- Is remaining childless an option, and if so, what ministry would fill the void?
- Are you willing to be a family without children?

Your Family Plan:

Peacekeeping Worksheet

FOR DECISIONS ABOUT:

Facts from Doctors or Tests

_____

_____

Facts from Research

_____

_____

Facts from Consultations

_____

_____

Doctors' Opinions and Suggestions

_____

_____

Input from Family/Friends/Mentors

_____

_____

Financial and Time Ramifications

_____

_____

Time with God in Prayer and Reading the Bible

_____

_____

Discussion Together of Thoughts, Opinions, and Desires

_____

_____

Our Peace-Filled Decision Is:

_____

_____

_____

_____

_____

Infertility Journey Map

On the "Milestone" lines, write in your Family Plan and the projected dates, then check off or highlight each milestone you pass. You'll begin feeling a sense of accomplishment and encouragement, and you'll have an overview of the journey you're traveling.

GIVE ME YOUR LANTERN AND COMPASS, GIVE ME A MAP SO I CAN FIND
MY WAY TO THE SACRED MOUNTAIN, TO THE PLACE OF YOUR PRESENCE,
TO ENTER THE PLACE OF WORSHIP, MEET MY EXUBERANT GOD, SING MY
THANKS WITH A HARP, MAGNIFICENT GOD, MY GOD.

(Ps. 43:3–4 *The Message*)

Milestone	Date
☐	
☐	
☐	
☐	
☐	
☐	
☐	
☐	
☐	
☐	
☐	
☐	
☐	
☐	
☐	
☐	
☐	
☐	
☐	
☐	
☐	

Appointment Notes

Appointment with:_____ Date:_____ Time:_____ Place:_____

Purpose of appointment:_____

_____

Question to ask:_____

_____

_____

Answer:_____

_____

_____

Question to ask:_____

_____

_____

Answer:_____

_____

_____

Question to ask:_____

_____

_____

Answer:_____

_____

_____

Question to ask:_____

_____

_____

Answer:_____

_____

_____

Information and instructions:_____

_____

_____

_____

_____

Phone Notes

Date:_____Time:_____ A.M./P.M._Who called:_____
Message:_____
_____

My response to the call:_____
_____

Date:_____Time:_____ A.M./P.M._Who called:_____
Message:_____
_____

My response to the call:_____
_____

Date:_____Time:_____ A.M./P.M._Who called:_____
Message:_____
_____

My response to the call:_____
_____

Date:_____Time:_____ A.M./P.M._Who called:_____
Message:_____
_____

My response to the call:_____
_____

Date:_____Time:_____ A.M./P.M._Who called:_____
Message:_____
_____

My response to the call:_____
_____

Date:_____Time:_____ A.M./P.M._Who called:_____
Message:_____
_____

My response to the call:_____
_____
_____
_____

Important Contact Information

Hospital_____
Address_____
Phone_____Billing Phone_____
Emergency Room Phone_____

Emergency Phone Numbers
Fire Department_____Police_____
Ambulance_____Paramedics_____

Pharmacy_____Pharmacist_____
Address_____
Phone_____After-Hours Phone_____
Delivery Available_____

Treatment Center_____
Address_____
Phone_____Billing Phone_____
Contact Person_____Ext._____

Counselor/Support Groups
Name of Agency_____E-mail_____
Address_____
Phone_____Meeting Times_____
Services They Provide_____
Contact Person_____

Home Health Services
Name of Agency_____
Address_____
Phone_____Nurse Case Manager_____
Nursing Services They Provide_____

Insurance Company_____
Address_____
Phone_____Policy Number_____
Group #_____Subscriber_____

Number_____ Web Site_____

Public Assistance #_____ Case Manager_____

Nutritional Assistance

Registered Dietitian_____ Phone_____

Location_____

Restaurants That Deliver_____

Transportation Services

Taxi Phone_____

Shuttle Services _____ Phone _____

Private Ride Services _____ Phone _____

Transportation Ministries _____ Phone_____

Church _____

Pastor _____ Phone _____ E-mail _____

Prayer Chain Number _____ Meals Ministry _____

Support Group Contact _____ Phone _____

Family and Friends

Name_____ Phone_____ E-mail_____

Name_____ Phone_____ E-mail_____

Name_____ Phone_____ E-mail_____

Name_____ Phone_____ E-mail_____

Name_____ Phone_____ E-mail_____

Name_____ Phone_____ E-mail_____

Name_____ Phone_____ E-mail_____

Name_____ Phone_____ E-mail_____

Name_____ Phone_____ E-mail_____

Name_____ Phone_____ E-mail_____

Name_____ Phone_____ E-mail_____

Name_____ Phone_____ E-mail_____

Name_____ Phone_____ E-mail_____

Name_____ Phone_____ E-mail_____

Name_____ Phone_____ E-mail_____

Name_____ Phone_____ E-mail_____

Name_____ Phone_____ E-mail_____

Name_____ Phone_____ E-mail_____

Test Results

Date	Test Name	Results	Retest Date

Medication / Shots Record

Drug	Dose / Freq	Start / Stop	Reason	X When Taken

Your Support and Help Team

Name_____ Home Phone_____
Work Phone_____ Cell Phone_____
Address_____ E-mail_____
How could this person help me?_____
_____
_____
_____

What did they offer to do?_____
_____
_____
_____

Name_____ Home Phone_____
Work Phone_____ Cell Phone_____
Address_____ E-mai_____
How could this person help me?_____
_____
_____
_____

What did they offer to do?_____
_____
_____

Name_____ Home Phone_____
Work Phone_____ Cell Phone_____
Address_____ E-mail_____
How could this person help me?_____
_____
_____
_____

What did they offer to do?_____
_____
_____

Bless You! Here's Where I Need Help

- ☐ Rides:
  - ☐ When
  - ☐ Where
  - ☐ How Long It Will Take
- ☐ Meals:
  - ☐ Breakfast
  - ☐ Lunch
  - ☐ Dinner
- ☐ Shopping:
  - ☐ Groceries
  - ☐ Medications
  - ☐ Personal Items
  - ☐ Other
- ☐ Child Care:
  - ☐ What Days?
  - ☐ What Hours?
  - ☐ Your Home
  - ☐ My Home
- ☐ "Me" Care:
  - ☐ What Hours?
  - ☐ Your Home
  - ☐ My Home
- ☐ Rides for the Kids (Specify days and times):
  - ☐ School
  - ☐ Sports
  - ☐ Church

- ☐ Activities
- ☐ Other
- ☐ Prayer Partners
- ☐ Someone to Call When I Am Down
- ☐ Someone to Call When I Am Up
- ☐ Housecleaning
- ☐ Laundry
- ☐ Answering E-mails
- ☐ Sending Thank-You Notes
- ☐ Running Errands
- ☐ Taking Over Some Commitments I Have at Church or on a Committee
- ☐ Filling In for Me at Work
- ☐ Accompany Me to Doctors' Appointments
- ☐ Go Shopping with Me to Buy Baby Things for a Quick Adoption
- ☐ _____
- ☐ _____
- ☐ _____
- ☐ _____

Stages of Grief

I wholeheartedly believe that without my relationship with God, I wouldn't be here right now because my grief would have been too overwhelming. Instead, I decided I wasn't going to let grief define me. You can't go around grief; the more you run from it, the more it comes after you. So I decided to meet it head-on. It wasn't easy, but I believe I'm a better person for having grabbed it by the horns and held on until I was ready to let go, instead of grief being a constant burden on my shoulders. —Sarah

Go through the following stages in the grieving process at your own pace, but keep moving. Check off your progress.

- ☐ *Shock* is the first reaction. The punch or sinking sensation in the pit of your stomach—dizzying, nauseating, room-spinning, unbelievable!
- ☐ *Denial* is a survival reaction until you get your bearings. You think, "This can't be happening to me." You hold on to the possibility it's all a mistake and try ignoring it.
- ☐ *Acknowledgment* replaces denial. Now you must face it head-on, and it hurts so bad and makes you so mad!
- ☐ *Anger* often is intense. Maybe you aren't angered easily, but now you are *angry*—angry with yourself, genetics, your circumstances, and maybe even God.
- ☐ *Acceptance* results from anger because you can't be angry at something you haven't accepted.
- ☐ *Sadness* seeps in as the dust settles on anger and the emotional and physical pain of acceptance engulfs you.
- ☐ *Depression* is the deepest form of sadness and can become debilitating and dangerous if you don't take steps to move through it.
- ☐ *Joy* can be the aftermath of healthy grieving. With prayer, support, counsel, and time, God says, "You will grieve, but your grief will suddenly turn to wonderful joy when you see me again" (John 16:20 NLT).

Signs of Depression

Finally, after dealing with these symptoms for a year, I went to our family doctor and was diagnosed with depression. In retrospect, I was naïve about that medical condition. When I was given the list of depression symptoms, I discovered I had every one, except suicidal thoughts. Infertility had finally taken its toll. Depression made me question everything about religion and faith and broke my heart beyond recognition. —Sharon

SHARON'S SYMPTOMS OF DEPRESSION

- ☐ Began shutting down physically and emotionally
- ☐ Started sleeping more and eating less
- ☐ Didn't cry for an entire year
- ☐ Ability to concentrate was impaired and couldn't make decisions
- ☐ Felt mentally weak
- ☐ Anxiety progressed to panic attacks
- ☐ Every aspect of life was suspended, as if in slow motion
- ☐ Took lots of sick days from work
- ☐ Lost interest in all hobbies
- ☐ Became agitated and panicked at seeing or hearing a baby or child

LIST OF MAJOR DEPRESSION SYMPTOMS COMPILED BY MAYO CLINIC
www.mayoclinic.com/health/depression/DS00175/DSECTION=symptoms

- ☐ Feelings of sadness or unhappiness
- ☐ Irritability or frustration, even over small matters
- ☐ Loss of interest or pleasure in normal activities
- ☐ Reduced sex drive
- ☐ Insomnia or excessive sleeping
- ☐ Changes in appetite—decreased appetite and weight loss, but can also cause increased food cravings and weight gain
- ☐ Agitation or restlessness—pacing, hand-wringing, or an inability to sit still
- ☐ Slowed thinking, speaking, or body movements
- ☐ Indecisiveness, distractibility, and decreased concentration
- ☐ Fatigue, tiredness, and loss of energy—even small tasks seem to require a lot of effort
- ☐ Feelings of worthlessness or guilt, fixating on past failures or blaming yourself when things aren't going right
- ☐ Trouble thinking, concentrating, making decisions, and remembering
- ☐ Frequent thoughts of death, dying, or suicide
- ☐ Crying spells for no apparent reason
- ☐ Unexplained physical problems, such as back pain or headaches

For some, symptoms are so severe it's obvious something isn't right. Others feel generally miserable or unhappy without really knowing why. Depression affects each person in different ways, so depression symptoms vary from person to person. Inherited traits, age, gender, and cultural background all play a role in how depression may affect you.

Ten Ways to Survive the Holidays When You're Infertile

Laura Christenson, a Mommy-in-Waiting and author of *The Adoption Decision*

If the mere thought of babies being handled by fawning relatives is enough to make you burst into tears and run for cover, try the following alternatives. You'll survive the holidays, and you may even celebrate them joyfully and triumphantly.

1. **Take charge.** Organize a party for the childless couples and singles in your church. Craft clay ornaments, decorate sugar cookies, or make wreaths.
2. **Just say "No."** Graciously decline invitations to child-oriented events. Send a note or gift to the hosts, letting them know how much you appreciate them.
3. **Pray.** If you plan to share the holidays with extended family or friends, pray for patience, wisdom, and strength. Contact a trusted family member before your arrival and schedule a leisurely walk together during the party.
4. **Send cards from Kitty.** Write a holiday newsletter from the perspective of your cat, dog, cockatoo, or hamster. Detail the events of your pet's year. Include photos of your pet, jauntily clad in holiday attire.
5. **Run away from home.** Take a mini vacation with your spouse to a romantic bed and breakfast inn. Make your marriage—not your baby quest—top priority during this time. Remind each other that it doesn't take a child to make a family; you and your spouse are a family already.
6. **Learn a winter sport together.** Cross-country ski, ice skate, or snowshoe. They're inexpensive, relatively safe, and emotionally refreshing.
7. **Get crafty.** Create handmade greeting cards, design jewelry, or construct wooden paper towel holders. Sell them at a holiday bazaar.
8. **Serve selflessly.** Spend a day serving at the local soup kitchen, mission, or shelter.
9. **Wax poetic.** Compose a romantic song or poem for your spouse. On Christmas morning, perform your masterpiece.
10. **Write a love letter to God.** Thank him for giving you life and for loving you more than you can comprehend. Ask him to guide you through this difficult time. God is always there to listen, and he understands.

You have an opportunity to do #10 at the end of each chapter in this book.

Infertility–Satan's Lies and God's Truths

Compiled by Sarah Cochran, a contributing Mommy-in-Waiting

Satan's Lies	God's Truths
If God loved me, I wouldn't be suffering from infertility; he doesn't care that my heart is broken.	We do not know what we ought to pray for, but the Spirit himself intercedes for us with groans that words cannot express. (Romans 8:26b) Psalm 66:10 Romans 5:3–5 Lamentations 3:22 1 Peter 4:12 Luke 12:7a
I don't need to rest in order to heal; I don't need to stop and refuel.	Then, because so many people were coming and going that they did not even have a chance to eat, [Jesus] said to them, "Come with me by yourselves to a quiet place and get some rest." (Mark 6:31) Psalm 46:10 Mark 6:46 Psalm 62:5 John 11:54
I don't understand why God is letting this happen.	"For my thoughts are not your thoughts, neither are your ways my ways," declares the LORD. (Isaiah 55:8) Job 28:23–24 Ecclesiastes 11:5
I'm not strong enough to endure this; life isn't supposed to be this hard.	The Lord is my rock, my fortress and my deliverer; my God is my rock in whom I take refuge, my shield and the horn of my salvation. He is my stronghold, my refuge and my savior. (2 Samuel 22:2–3a) Job 2:10b Psalm 22:19 Psalm 9:9 2 Corinthians 12:9–10
I'll be in this hole forever; there's no way out.	He lifted me out of the slimy pit, out of the mud and mire; he set my feet on a rock and gave me a firm place to stand. (Psalm 40:2) Psalm 18:16 2 Corinthians 4:16–18
I am all alone.	When you pass through the waters, [God] will be with you; and when you pass through the rivers, they will not sweep over you. When you walk through the fire, you will not be burned; the flames will not set you ablaze. (Isaiah 43:2) Joshua 1:9b Psalm 40:1–3a Psalm 38:15 Hebrews 13:5b
I have a right to stay angry; I don't need to forgive others; they don't deserve my forgiveness.	Get rid of all bitterness, rage and anger, brawling and slander, along with every form of malice. Be kind and compassionate to one another, forgiving each other, just as in Christ God forgave you. (Ephesians 4:31–32) Mark 11:25 Luke 23:34a Luke 6:37c Colossians 3:13

God let me down; he got it wrong; I can't trust him; I can't forgive him.	Let us hold unswervingly to the hope we profess, for he [God] who promised is faithful. (Hebrews 10:23) Job 2:10b John 11:4b Proverbs 3:5–6 2 Corinthians 10:5 Nahum 1:7
God can't ease my burden of hurt; my hurt is too big for him.	Come to me [Jesus], all you who are weary and burdened, and I will give you rest. (Matthew 11:28) Psalm 147:3 Peter 5:7 2 Corinthians 1:3b–4a Revelation 7:17c
My hurt is so overwhelming that I can't praise God; it's too hard.	This is what the Lord, the God of your father David, says: I have heard your prayers and seen your tears; I will heal you. (2 Kings 20:5b) Job 13:15a Psalm 126:5 Psalm 43:5 John 16:20
I have no hope; God can't comfort me.	I pray also that the eyes of your heart may be enlightened in order that you may know the hope to which he has called you, the riches of his glorious inheritance in the saints. (Ephesians 1:18) Job 11:18 Jeremiah 31:17a Psalm 116:8–9 Micah 7:7 Psalm 130:5 Romans 15:13 Proverbs 23:18
God has forgotten me.	But the needy will not always be forgotten, nor the hope of the afflicted ever perish. (Psalm 9:18) Isaiah 38:5 Jeremiah 29:11–14a Isaiah 41:10
I'll never stop crying.	The Sovereign Lord will wipe away the tears from all faces. (Isaiah 25:8b) Psalm 147:3 Psalm 30:5b Revelation 21:4a
I'd be better off without God.	For in the day of trouble [God] will keep me safe in his dwelling; he will hide me in the shelter of his tabernacle and set me high upon a rock. (Psalm 27:5) Psalm 32:7 Psalm 84:10
I don't need to share my story with others.	Always be prepared to give an answer to everyone who asks you to give the reason for the hope that you have. (1 Peter 3:15b) 2 Corinthians 1:4

Prayer & Praise Journal

The best Sanity Tool is a place to write specific prayer requests and then record the answers. After you've written your requests to God, return and make a notation of the day and way he answered. When you're having a bad day, read these pages and see God in action. Revisit your journal on good days so you remember the source of your joy.

Psalm 77:1 *The Message*

I yell out to my God, I yell with all my might, I yell at the top of my lungs. He listens.

Psalm 77:11–12 *The Message*

Once again I'll go over what GOD has done, lay out on the table the ancient wonders; I'll ponder all the things you've accomplished, and give a long, loving look at your acts.

Prayer Request	Praise